J. HART

A.P. 3125

PRINCIPLES OF ANATOMY AND PHYSIOLOGY FOR PHYSICAL TRAINING INSTRUCTORS IN THE ROYAL AIR FORCE

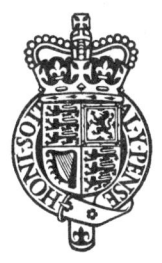

LONDON
HER MAJESTY'S STATIONERY OFFICE
1959

Price £1 3s 0d [£1·15] net

First published . . 1946
Third edition . . . 1959
Fourth impression . . 1970

© *Crown copyright* 1959

Published by
Her Majesty's Stationery Office

To be purchased from
49 High Holborn, London w.c.1
13a Castle Street, Edinburgh eh2 3ar
109 St. Mary Street, Cardiff cf1 1jw
Brazennose Street, Manchester m60 8as
50 Fairfax Street, Bristol bs1 3de
258 Broad Street, Birmingham 1
7 Linenhall Street, Belfast bt2 8ay
or through any bookseller

First Promulgated by Command of the Air Council

MINISTRY OF DEFENCE

By Command of the Defence Council
Henry Hardman

Air Publication 3125

The amendments promulgated in the undermentioned list have been made in this publication.

| Amendment List || Amendments made by | Date |
Number	Date		

CONTENTS

Chapter			Page
	FOREWORD		vii
	FOREWORD TO SECOND EDITION		viii
	FOREWORD TO THIRD EDITION		ix
I	ANATOMY	1 The Bony Framework	1
		2 Joints	17
		3 The Muscular System	28
II	PHYSIOLOGY	1 The Vascular System	91
		2 The Respiratory System	96
		3 The Alimentary System	100
		4 The Excretory System	106
		5 The Nervous System	107
		6 Muscular Action	114
III	POSTURE AND CORRECTIVE EXERCISES		118
IV	BREATHING		135
V	FITNESS FOR FLYING		140
VI	GENERAL FITNESS		144
VII	MEDICAL REHABILITATION		149

FOREWORD

THE purpose of this manual is to explain certain important principles of anatomy and physiology which are particularly related to physical fitness.

It should be the aim of every instructor in physical fitness to know these basic principles because, with such knowledge, he will have a better understanding of the application of exercises and an increased interest in his work. In addition, he will have more confidence in discussing with the medical staff any difficult points which may arise. It is only by well balanced co-operation between the Medical and Physical Training Branches that the best results can be obtained.

Emphasis is laid on the functional rather than the theoretical aspect of anatomy, and the sections on physiology present only certain aspects of this subject.

In Chapters III, IV and VII, importance is attached to the reason for any particular exercise rather than to the specific method of carrying it out; no attempt therefore is made to set out detailed lists of exercises.

Chapter V deals with mental and physical fatigue and fitness for flying, and presents a brief outline of methods used to overcome certain difficulties which an instructor is likely to encounter when working with flying personnel.

Chapter VI gives a brief outline of methods useful for preserving general health and fitness among all types of personnel on Royal Air Force stations.

Chapter VII deals with the rehabilitation of medical and surgical cases and describes the general methods and grading of remedial activity. The importance of the psychological factor in patients who have been long in hospital is stressed, as well as their need for careful and individual handling. Instructors should understand that, as they are dealing with men in varying stages of recovery from injury and illness, their work in a rehabilitation centre is under the close guidance of the medical officer, whereas at a Royal Air Force station, the supervision of physical activities is left largely in their hands.

The last part of this chapter contains a short description of some of the common pathological conditions seen at Rehabilitation Centres.

H. E. WHITTINGHAM,
Director-General of Medical Services

Air Ministry,
May, 1945

FOREWORD TO SECOND EDITION

THIS edition of the Principles of Anatomy and Physiology for Physical Training Instructors in the Royal Air Force represents a thorough revision of the original text. Errors of fact and statements of doubtful validity have been corrected or omitted and some passages have been entirely rewritten. I wish to acknowledge the valuable assistance given by Professor F. Wood Jones, F.R.C.S., F.R.S. and Dr. F. S. Gorrill, M.D., M.R.C.P., of the Department of Anatomy of the Royal College of Surgeons of England who were so kind as to revise the text and to recommend alterations where they considered them to be necessary.

P. C. LIVINGSTON
Director-General of Medical Services

Air Ministry,
July, 1949

FOREWORD TO THE THIRD EDITION

THE publication of this third edition of the Principles of Anatomy and Physiology for Physical Training Instructors has called for but little alteration of the original text.

There have been a few minor amendments in the Physiology Chapter in relation to muscle tone.

Chapter III on "Posture and Corrective Exercises" has been revised, eliminating statements of doubtful validity and altering the emphasis to be more in keeping with current practice.

Chapter VII on "Medical Rehabilitation" has been completely rewritten. As the training of P.T.Is. for work in rehabilitation units has now been incorporated with the syllabus of training for remedial Gymnasts, a cursory survey of the principles of remedial work and the section on the "Elementary Pathology of Conditions Commonly Seen at Rehabilitation Centres" no longer has a place in this Manual. However, as remedial gymnastics is an important specialisation for Physical Training Instructors, a brief description of medical rehabilitation units, their personnel and work has been included.

The chapter on "Questions Commonly Asked by Instructors" has been deleted as it has been found that questions of this nature are best dealt with directly in the light of current informed opinions.

P. B. LEE POTTER
Director-General of Medical Services

Air Ministry,
May, 1959

CHAPTER I
ANATOMY
SECTION 1—THE BONY FRAMEWORK

Before describing the skeleton, it is first necessary to say a little about the nature of the material of which its various parts are composed and then to describe general types of bones, divided according to their function in the body.

Bone

Bone is a substance which provides the body with a rigid supporting framework and it is specially adapted to withstand mechanical stress and strain; at the same time, its weight, compared with its strength, is small. It is composed of a lime salt (calcium phosphate) deposited in a network of very strong fibres. The lime gives rigidity to the bone, while the fibrous network makes it resilient; a bone without this resilience would be brittle and much more liable to fracture. More lime is deposited in the bone as we grow older, and it is for this reason that fractures are so apt to occur from minor injuries as age increases.

Two kinds of bone are found in the skeleton:

(1) a hard, dense substance called *compact* bone; this forms the surface layer of the bone and provides the necessary rigidity. The blood supply of compact bone is maintained by numerous small vessels which pierce the surface and permeate its substance.

(2) a soft somewhat spongy substance called *cancellous* bone; it forms a lattice work structure between the compact outer walls; in its interstices it contains the *marrow*. Marrow may be either red or yellow in colour; in long bones, such as the shin bone, it is yellow; in flat bones, for example, the shoulder blade, it is red. It consists of numerous blood cells, special marrow cells and fat cells; it provides the material for the repair of fractures and also manufactures some of the cells of the blood.

The surface of every bone is closely covered by a strong membrane called the *periosteum*; it is richly supplied with blood vessels and acts as a medium through which the bone receives a large part of its blood supply; for this reason it plays a very important part in the repair of fractures.

Cartilage

Cartilage, commonly known as gristle, is pale, blue-white in colour and of firm but elastic consistence; though it can resist a considerable compressing force, it is of low tensile strength and can be cut quite easily with a knife. It is found in various parts of the body, for example, in the ears, nose, ribs, and in the joints where it is necessary to have rigidity and strength combined with elasticity.

Its main functions are to act as:

(1) a temporary framework for the bones and joints of children, being gradually replaced by bone as they become older. The fact that fractures are relatively rare among children in spite of frequent heavy falls, is due to the large proportion of cartilage present in their skeletal framework.

(2) a lining to the joints between bones, increasing the accuracy of the fitting together of joint surfaces.

(3) a resilient support between bony structures to lessen the forces of shock which may be applied.

Ligament

A ligament is a collection of tough white fibres compactly fitted together to form a cord or band. Its special function is to hold bony structures together and to withstand tension; ligaments have almost no elasticity* but may become stretched under prolonged strain.

General Types of Bones

For the present purpose, only five types of bones need be considered; these are:

(1) the cancellous, segmental bone;
(2) the long, heavy bone;
(3) the flat, thin bone;
(4) the long, thin bone;
(5) the small, compact bone.

A typical example of the first kind of bone is one of the bones of the back, called a *vertebra* (Figure 1). Its main function is that of support, and it makes joints with the adjacent vertebrae for movement of the vertebral column as a whole.

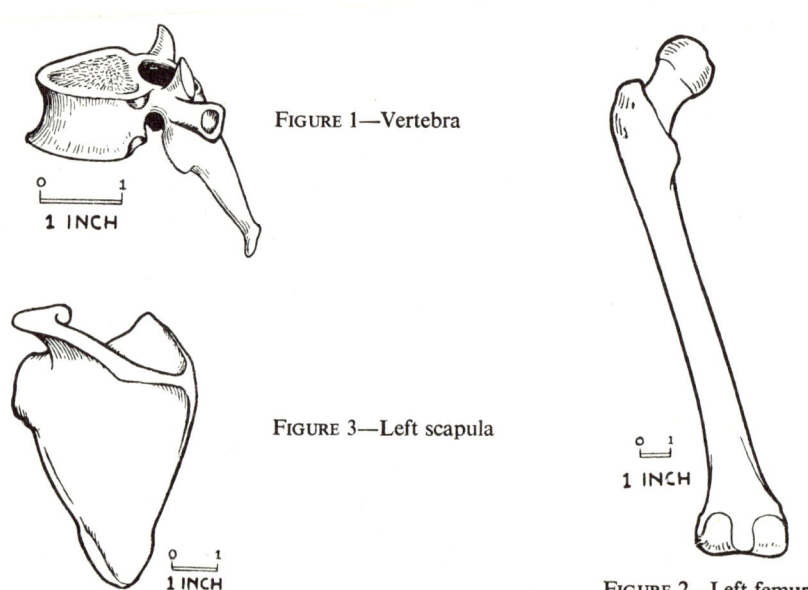

FIGURE 1—Vertebra

FIGURE 3—Left scapula

FIGURE 2—Left femur

An example of the second type, the long, heavy bone, is the thigh-bone or *femur* (Figure 2); it is specially built to bear weight and provides a large surface at each end for strong joints.

The shoulder blade or *scapula* (Figure 3) is an example of a flat thin bone; its main function is to provide broad surfaces for the attachment of muscles.

*There is a special type of ligament found between the bones of the spine which is yellow in colour and very elastic to allow spinal movement to take place.

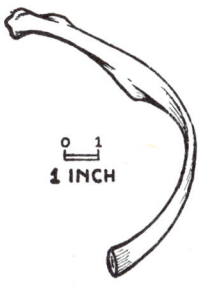
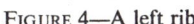
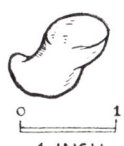

FIGURE 5—The left scaphoid

FIGURE 4—A left rib

A *rib* is an example of the fourth type, the long thin bone; its main function is to supply a moving framework (Figure 4).

The fifth type is the small compact bone which is rather like a pebble; the example shown is one of the bones of the wrist (Figure 5). Their main function is to supply the flexibility and strength necessary for the movement of the hands and feet.

THE SKELETON

The skeleton consists of the skull, the backbone, the ribs, the shoulder girdle, the bones of the upper limbs, the pelvis and the bones of the lower limbs.

The anatomy of the skull does not come within the scope of this book.

The Vertebral Column or Backbone (Figure 6)

The vertebral column is divided into regions:

(1) *cervical* or neck;
(2) *dorsal* or back;
(3) *lumbar* or loin;
(4) *sacral* or rump;
(5) *coccygeal* or tail.

There are seven units, or vertebrae, in the cervical region, twelve in the dorsal five in the lumbar; five are fused together in the sacral region to form one bone, the *sacrum*. The four small bones fused to form the *coccyx* are the remnant of the tail and serve to remind us of man's humble origin.

The vertebral column is the structure through which the weight of the upper part of the body is transmitted to the lower limbs.

There are two curves in the column which develop soon after birth, the *cervical* and *lumbar*; both curves are convex forward. The cervical curve appears when the child begins to hold up its head; the lumbar curve starts to develop when the erect position is adopted, and is at first exaggerated, giving rise to the normal hollow back and protruding abdomen of very young children but at the age of three or four, when the abdominal musculature become better developed, it assumes its adult shape.

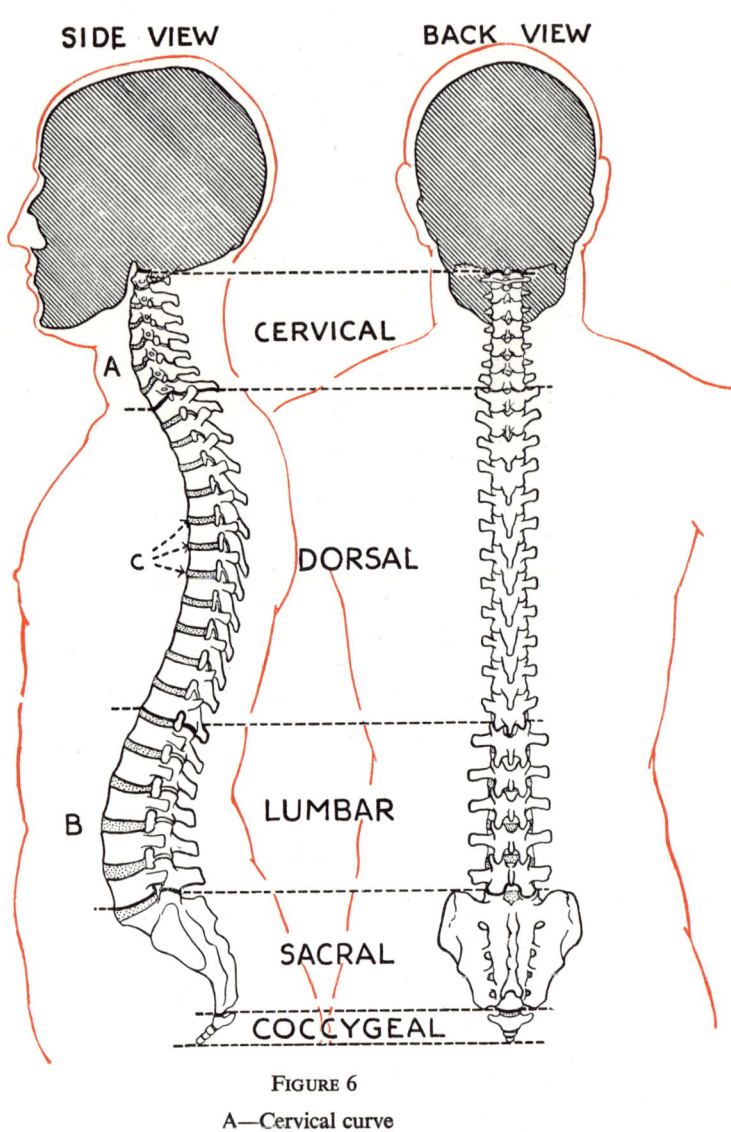

FIGURE 6
A—Cervical curve
B—Lumbar curve
C—Intervertebral discs

The Invertebral Discs

A thick pad of fibrous, elastic tissue, called an *intervertebral* disc lies between one vertebra and another. These discs serve a dual purpose;

(1) they act as shock absorbers, allowing a limited amount of movement between adjacent vertebrae;

(2) they assist in maintaining the shape of the vertebral column, and make up about one quarter of its total length.

A Typical Vertebra (Figure 7)

A typical vertebra, for example a dorsal vertebra, is composed of a body a strong arch, four small bony processes called facets, two transverse processes and a spinous process.

The body consists of a mass of cancellous bone, the upper and lower surfaces of which are flattened; the depth of the body is approximately one inch, the front and sides are rounded.

The arch of bone project backwards from the body and gives protection to the spinal cord which passes between it and the body of the vertebra.

Two of the facets project upward and two project downward. These facets arise from the bases of the pillars of the arch and articulate* with the corresponding facets on the vertebrae above and below; the joints so formed allow very slight up and down and side to side movement but the aggregate of these movements in the whole vertebral column is considerable.

The transverse processes are small finger-like structures projecting outward from each side of the arch. The spinous process projects backward and downward from the top of the arch. These three processes provide surfaces for the attachments of the muscles of the back and act as powerful levers for spinal movements.

*Articulate means to form a joint.

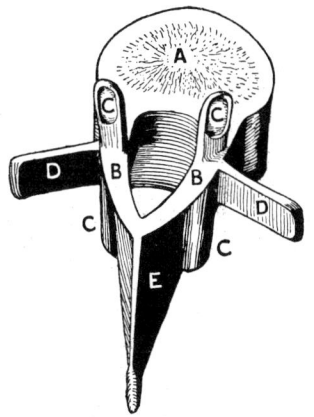

FIGURE 7—Diagram of a typical vertebra
   A—Body   C—Articular facet
   B—Arch   D—Transverse process
     E—Spinous process

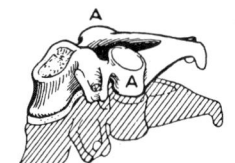

FIGURE 8—Cervical vertebra
   A—Articular facet

The shape, size and structure of the vertebrae vary according to their position in the vertebral column; from the neck downward they become larger and more solid.

The Cervical Vertebrae (Figure 8)

The cervical vertebrae, with the exception of the first two, which have special characteristics and which will be described later, are smaller than either the dorsal or lumbar vertebrae, and their articular facets are shaped to allow a greater range of rotation thereby increasing the field of vision and making it nearly possible for man to see behind him.

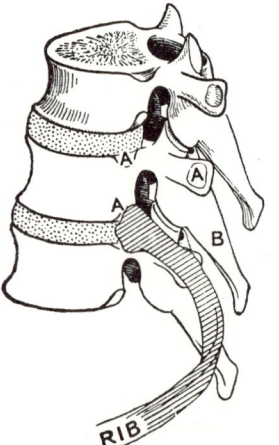

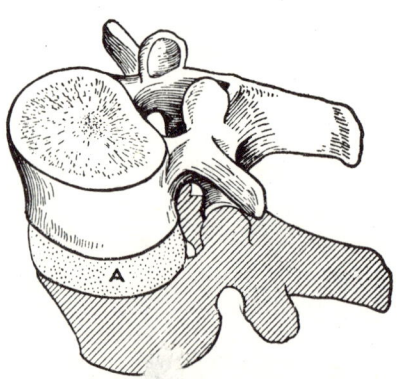

FIGURE 9—Dorsal vertebrae
    A—Articular surface for rib
    B—Spinous process

FIGURE 10—Lumbar vertebrae
    A—Intervertebral disc

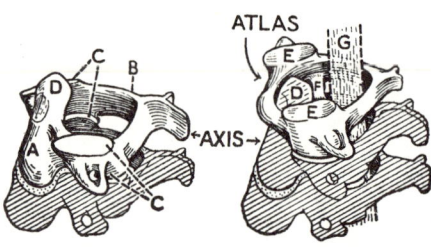

FIGURE 11—The axis and atlas
- A—Body
- B—Arch
- C—Articular facet
- D—Vertical peg
- E—Articular facet for skull
- F—Ligament
- G—Spinal cord

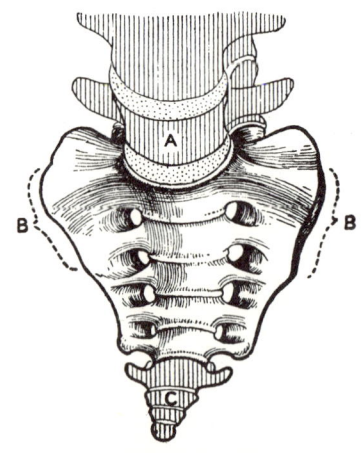

FIGURE 12—Sacrum and coccyx, front view
    A—Fifth lumbar vertesra
    B—Articular surface for hip bone
    C—Coccyx

The Dorsal Vertebrae (Figure 9)

The dorsal vertebrae have small articular surfaces on the bodies and transverse processes for atriculation with the ribs, which make joints with them on each side. Their spinous processes are longer than those of the other vertebrae and overlie one another closely, in this way preventing too much backward movement in the dorsal region.

The Lumbar Vertebrae (Figure 10)

The lumbar vertebrae are very much larger and stronger than the dorsal or cervical vertebrae. For example, in the adult man, the width of the body of the fifth lumbar vertebra, the largest in the vertebral column, is approximately two inches, while that of the body of the third cervical (Figure 8) is not more than half an inch.

The size and strength of the intervertebral discs, which lie between the vertebrae, are also increased progressively down the spine, so that they may withstand the greater weight and strain to which they are subjected.

The Axis (Figure 11)

The second cervical vertebra called the *axis* will, for the sake of convenience, be described first; it is a ring-shaped vertebra consisting of a small body, a fairly wide arch, two transverse and one spinous process for muscular attachments, and four articular facets one above and one below the base of each pillar of the arch. Its special characteristic, however, is a peg of bone which projects vertically upward from its body to articulate with the front portion of the first cervical vertebra, the *atlas*. This bony peg forms a vertical axis, as its name implies, round which the atlas and upon it, the head, can rotate in a horizontal plane.

The Atlas (Figure 11)

The *atlas*, so called because its action can be compared with that of the mythological Atlas who was thought to support the heavens upon his shoulders, is very similar in general structure to the axis, but its body has joined the axis to form the vertical peg.

The space in its centre is divided into two parts by a strong ligament; the front part of the space is occupied by the vertical bony process of the axis and the back part by the spinal cord. The ligament holds the bony process of the axis in position and prevents it from slipping backward and injuring the cord.

The Sacrum (Figure 12)

The five vertebrae which make up the sacrum are fused together in the shape of a concave wedge, the concavity of which faces forward.

It articulates above with the fifth lumbar vertebra and, at the sides, with the inner surfaces of the two hip or *innominate* bones, thus forming the posterior part of the pelvic girdle.

The Coccyx (Figure 12)

The coccyx is continuous with the lower part of the sacrum and serves chiefly as an attachment for muscles of the pelvic floor.

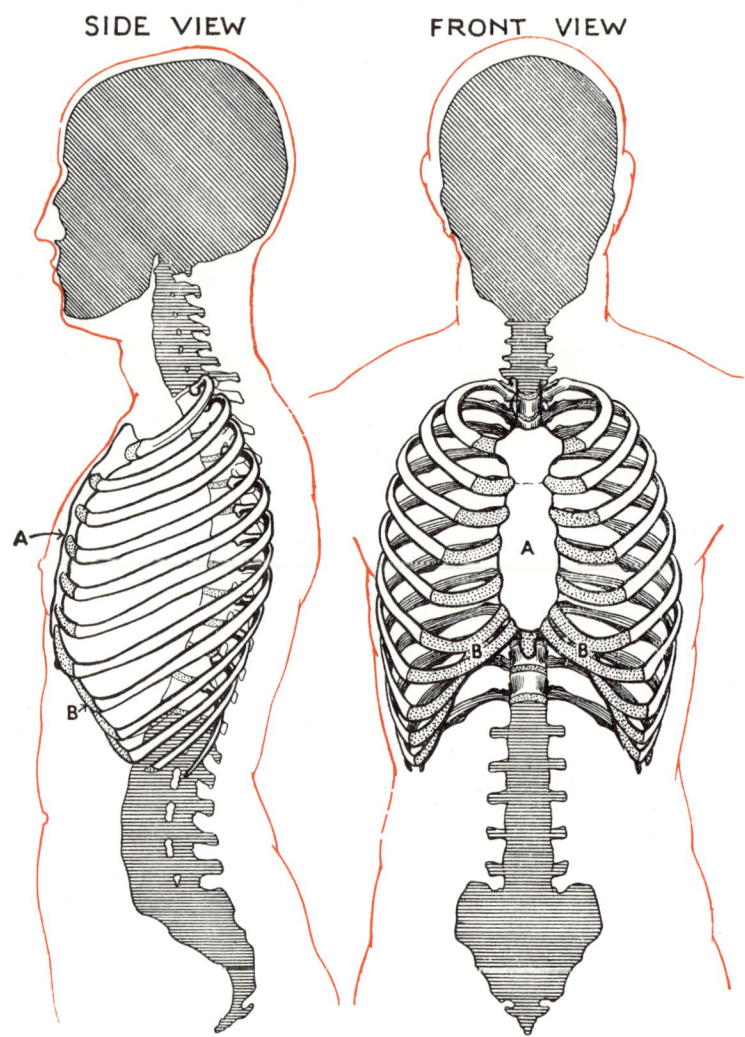

Figure 13—The thorax
A—Sternum
B—Costal cartilage

The Thorax (Figure 13)

The bones of the thorax make up a dome-shaped structure; they are the breast bone, or *sternum*, the twelve pairs of ribs and the twelve dorsal vertebrae.

Each rib is attached at the back to the body of the vertebra and the front of the transverse process. In front it is attached to the sternum by a length of cartilage called the *costal* cartilage. This cartilage gives the chest wall elasticity which makes possible the movements necessary for breathing.

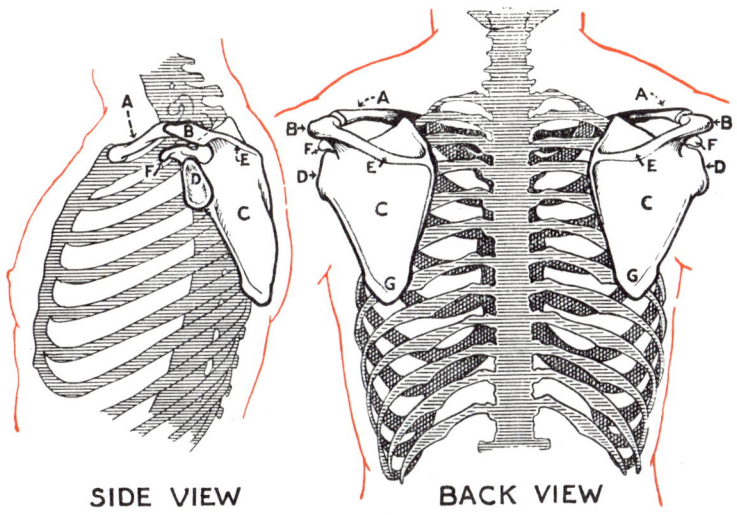

SIDE VIEW   BACK VIEW

FIGURE 14—The shoulder girdle
A—Clavicle   D—Glenoid fossa
B—Acromion   E—Spine of scapula
C—Scapula   F—Coracoid process
G—Inferior angle of scapula

The Upper Limbs

The bones of the upper limbs consist of the two collar bones or *clavicles* and the two shoulder blades or *scapulae*, which form the *shoulder girdle* (Figure 14), and the bones of the arms and hands (Figure 15).

The Shoulder Girdle (Figure 14)

The shoulder girdle is a structure that provides a strong, mobile base by which each of the upper limbs is attached to the trunk. It is not adapted for weight bearing like the pelvic girdle, but for the performances of complex movements.

The *clavicle* is about six inches long and is attached at its inner end to the sternum by a joint which allows a fairly free range of movement. Its outer end articulates with the inner aspect of the *acromion* which is described below.

The clavicle acts as a prop to maintain the scapula and upper limb at the correct distance from the chest wall. Fractures of this bone, due to a fall on the outstretched arm, are very common; fortunately they usually unite rapidly and without residual disability.

The *scapula* is a flat, triangular bone which, in the position of rest, covers an area on the back of the chest extending from the second to the seventh rib.

At its outer angle there is an oval surface, facing outward and about one inch in diameter, with which the head of the humerus articulates; this is the *glenoid fossa*.

Across the back of the triangular portion of the scapula runs a prominent ridge of bone, called the *spine* of the scapula which extends outward and overhangs the shoulder joint; this overhanging part is called the *acromion*.

The scapula, by its broad flat surface and wide muscle attachments, maintains a very strong purchase on the chest wall, so providing a firm basis upon which movements of the upper limb can take place.

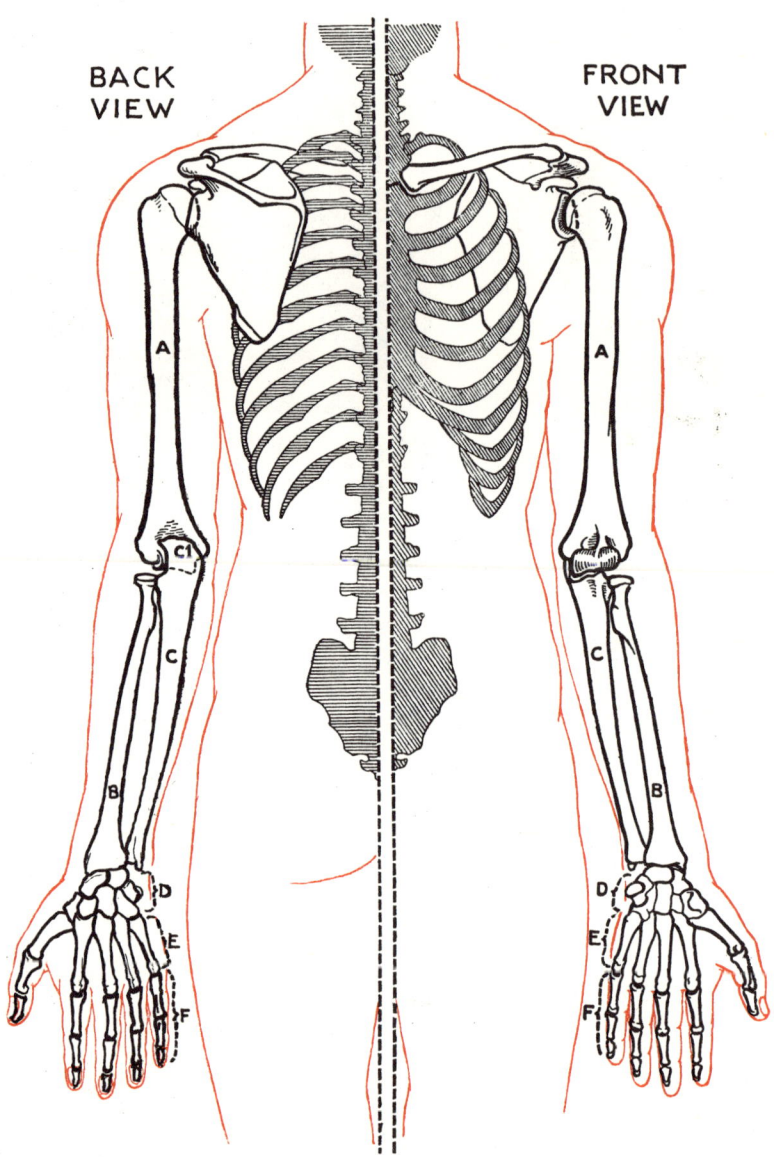

FIGURE 15—Skeleton of the arm and hand
A—Humerus D—Carpus
B—Radius E—Metacarpals
C—Ulna F—Phalanges
C^1—Olecranon

The Bones of the Arm and Hand (Figure 15)

The skeleton of the arm and hand consists of:
(1) the bone of the upper arm or *humerus*;
(2) the bones of the forearm, the *radius* and *ulna*;
(3) the eight small bones of the wrist forming the *carpus*;
(4) the nineteen bones of the fingers called *metacarpals* and *phalanges*.

The Humerus

The humerus is a long bone and consists of a head, a neck, a shaft and a lower extremity. The head, which is the shape of a half-sphere, articulates with the glenoid fossa of the scapula to form the shoulder joint; the lower end articulates with the *radius* and *ulna* bones to make the elbow joint.

The Radius

The radius is a long thin bone consisting of a head, neck, shaft and lower extremity. The head is shaped like a thick disc, and its upper surface has a shallow depression which articulates with the outer part of the lower extremity of the humerus; the sides of this disc articulate with the upper portion of the ulna.

The shaft of the radius is slightly curved; it lies on the outer side of the ulna when the palm faces forward, and across the ulna when the palm faces backward. Its lower end helps to form the wrist joint and also articulates with the lower end of the ulna.

The Ulna

The ulna consists of an upper extremity, a shaft and a lower extremity. The upper extremity has a crescent-shaped notch which articulates with the inner and posterior portion of the lower end of the humerus. The tip of the upper extremity is a beak-shaped process of bone called the *olecranon*. When the arm is extended, this process fits into a depression at the back of the lower end of the humerus, locking the elbow joint and preventing further extension.

As mentioned above, the ulna articulates with the radius at its upper and lower ends. Its lower extremity also forms part of the wrist joint.

The Carpus

The carpus consists of eight small pebble-like bones closely fitted together in two rows, four bones in each row; it provides a flexible yet firm basis upon which the muscles of the forearm and hand can exert themselves.

The upper end of the carpus has a smoothly rounded surface which articulates with the lower end of the radius and ulna to form the wrist joint.

The lower end of the carpus articulates with the upper extremities of the metacarpals.

The Metacarpals and Phalanges

The metacarpals are five in number; they have each a straight shaft and an upper and lower articular surface. The first metacarpal forms the bony support of the base of the thumb; the remaining four provide a framework for the palm of the hand; the lower ends of these bones articulate with the upper ends of the first row of phalanges to form the knuckle joints.

The phalanges are the bones of the fingers and thumb; there are three phalanges in each finger and two in the thumb.

The Lower Limbs

The bones of the lower limbs consist of two hip or innominate bones, which, with the sacrum, form the *pelvic girdle* (Figure 16) and the bones of the legs (Figure 17) and the feet (Figure 18).

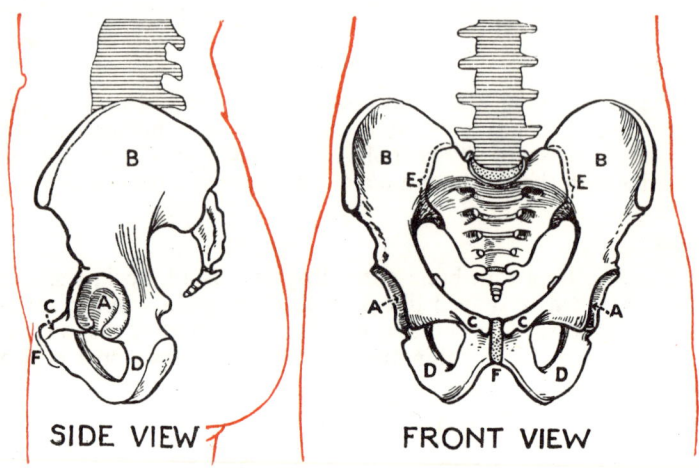

FIGURE 16—The pelvic girdle
A—Acetabulum   D—Ischium
B—Ilium   E—Sacro-iliac joints
C—Pubis   F—Pubic junction

The Pelvic Girdle (Figure 16)

In the middle portion of the outer side of each innominate bone, there is a deep socket called the *acetabulum*, which articulates with the head of the thigh bone or femur. The broad flat blade of bone above the acetabulum is called the *ilium*, the arch of bone below and in front of it the *pubis*, and the part below and behind, the *ischium*; the last forms the bony prominence in the buttock.

Each innominate bone is attached to the sacrum by strong ligaments, forming the *sacro-iliac* joints. In front, the two bones of the pubis are joined together to form a slightly movable joint, thus completing the pelvic girdle. In childbirth the ligaments supporting these joints become relaxed, allowing an increase in the size of the pelvic outlet.

The main function of the pelvis is to provide a solid base through which weight can be transmitted to the lower limbs from the upper part of the body; it also provides attachment for the very powerful muscles of the legs and lower part of the back.

The Bones of the Leg (Figure 17)

The skeleton of the leg consists of :

(1) the thigh bone or *femur*;

(2) the knee cap or *patella*;

(3) the shin bone or *tibia*;

(4) the brooch bone or *fibula* which is a long thin bone lying to the outer side of the tibia.

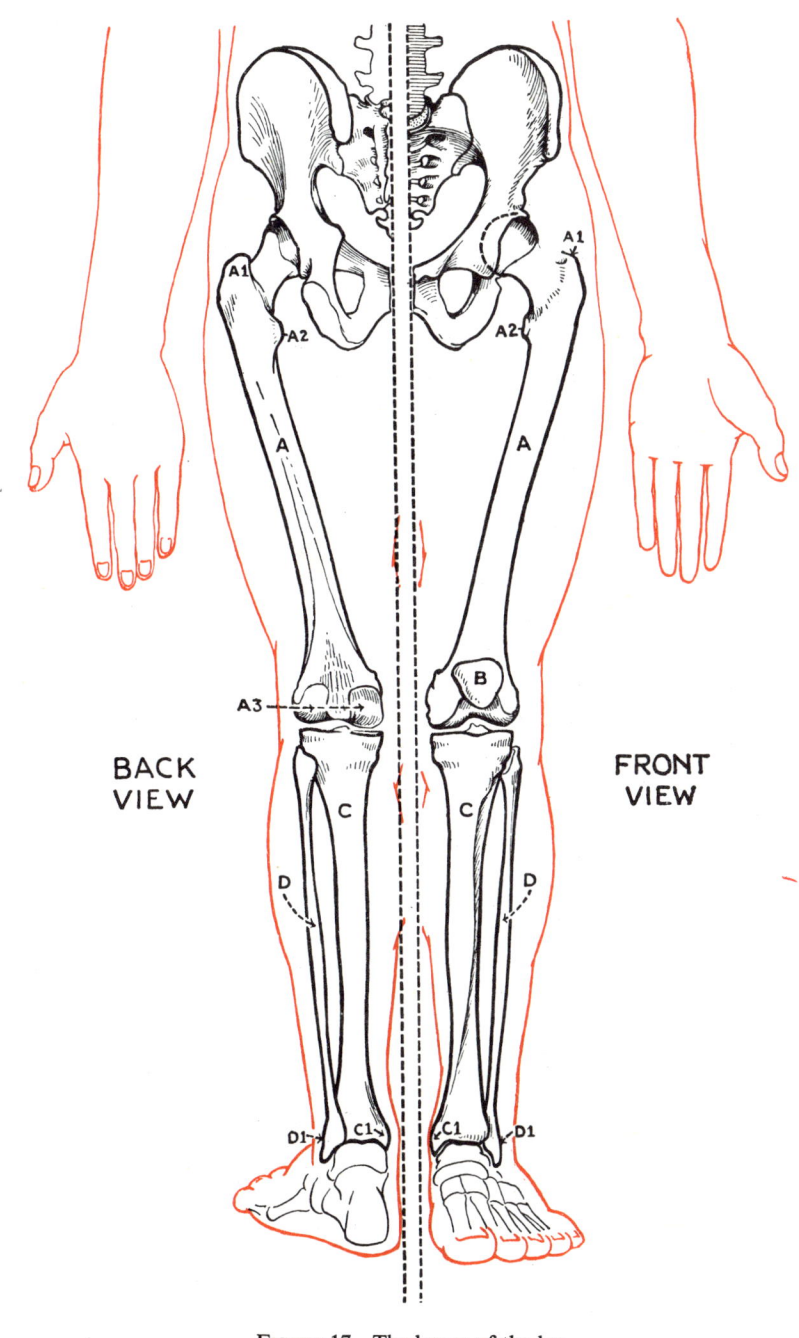

FIGURE 17—The bones of the leg

A—Femur
A¹—Greater trochanter
A²—Lesser trochanter
A³—Condyles
B—Patella
C—Tibia
C¹—Internal malleolus
D—Fibula
D¹—External malleolus

The Femur

The femur has a head, a neck, a shaft and a large lower extremity; it is the longest bone in the body. The head is spherical and articulates with the acetabulum. The neck is about an inch and a half in length, rounded and very strong; it joins the shaft of the femur at an angle of 125 degrees. The shaft has a slight forward convexity. A large bony prominence called the *greater trochanter*, projects from its upper extremity, and on the inner side of the shaft just below its neck, there is a small blunt spur of bone, the *lesser trochanter*. Certain important hip muscles are attached to these trochanters.

The shaft of the femur is directed slightly inward, forming an angle of about 170 degrees with the shaft of the tibia, when the body is in the upright position and the feet are together. The lower end of the shaft of the femur widens out to form two large articular surfaces called *condyles*, the inner condyle being slightly lower than the outer. These two condyles articulate with the upper end of the tibia to form the knee joint.

The Patella

The patella is situated in front of the knee joint in the tendon of the muscles which extend the knee. It is roughly circular in outline and about an inch and a half in diameter and half an inch thick; it has an inner and an outer surface; the inner surface articulates with the condyles of the femur. Its function is to improve leverage by its pulley like action as it glides in the groove between the smooth surfaces of the condyles. If the outer side of the groove is abnormally flat or if the angle between the shafts of the femur and tibia is considerably less than 170 degrees, the patella may dislocate to the outer side of the joint.

The Tibia

The tibia is so named on account of its likeness to the Roman flute; it has an upper and lower extremity and a shaft. The upper extremity provides a broad horizontal plateau which has an inner and an outer articular surface for the corresponding condyles of the femur. The shaft is straight and tapers slightly towards its lower end; it is triangular in cross-section. The lower extremity has a downward projection, the *internal malleolus*, on its inner side. The end of the shaft and the outer aspects of the internal malleolus form part of the ankle joint.

The Fibula

The fibula is a long, thin bone which has a head, shaft and lower extremity. Its head articulates with the outer side of the upper end of the tibia and its lower extremity is fixed by strong ligaments to the outer side of the lower end of the same bone. Its lower end, called the *external malleolus*, forms part of the ankle joint. The fibula does not transmit any weight, its main function being to supply a framework for muscle attachment and help to protect certain important blood vessels.

The Bones of the Foot (Figure 18)

The skeleton of the foot is made up of:
 (1) the seven bones of the main part of the foot which together make up the *tarsus*;
 (2) the five bones of the fore-foot called *metatarsals*;
 (3) the bones of the toes or *phalanges*.

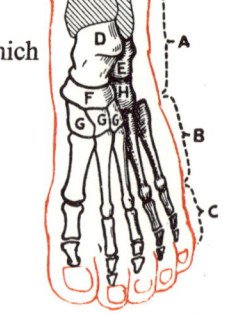

FIGURE 18—The skeleton of the foot
A—Tarsus   E—Calcaneus
B—Metatarsals   F—Navicular*
C—Phalanges   G—Cuneiform
D—Talus   H—Cuboid

TOP VIEW

*Navicular means boat-shaped.

The Tarsus

The two largest bones of the tarsus are the ankle bone or *talus*, sometimes called *astragalus*, and the heel bone, or *calcaneus*, sometimes called *os calcis*.

The upper surface of the talus articulates with the lower end of the tibia and fibula forming the ankle joint. The rounded surface on the front of the talus articulates with the *navicular* bone which in turn articulates with the three small *cuneiform* bones. The under surface of the talus makes three small joints with the upper surface of the calcaneus; the calcaneus, in addition to its articulation with the talus above it, forms a joint with the *cuboid* bone at its anterior extremity.

The Metatarsals and Phalanges

The metatarsals are similar in shape to the corresponding bones of the hand, but they are of greater size and strength. The upper ends of the inner three metatarsals articulate with the three cuneiform bones and the upper ends of the outer two with the cuboid bone.

The phalanges are generally shorter and thicker than those of the hand. There are two phalanges in the big toe and three in each of the remaining toes.

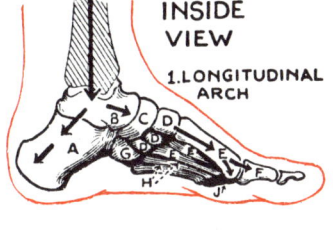
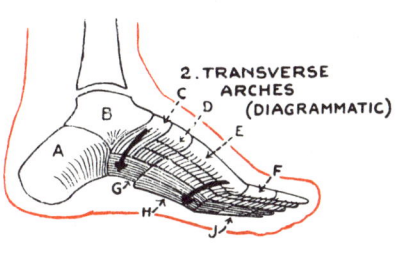

FIGURE 19—The longitudinal and transverse arches of the foot

A—Calcaneus
B—Talus
C—Navicular
D—Cuneiform
E—Inner three metatarsals
F—Phalanges of inner three toes
G—Cuboid
H—Outer two metatarsals
J—Phalanges of outer two toes

The Arches of the Foot (Figure 19)

Very great strains are imposed upon the feet, particularly during strenuous exercise. The foot is able to meet these strains because of the strength and flexibility of its structure. It is constructed in the form of arches which are held together by ligaments and supported by muscles. The arches are:

(1) longitudinal, extending from the heel to the toes:
(2) a series of transverse arches across the foot.

(1) The Longitudinal Arch

The longitudinal arch consists of an inner and an outer portion which rest on a common pillar behind, namely the calcaneus. The inner part of the longitudinal arch is formed by the calcaneus, the talus, the navicular, the three cuneiform bones and the inner three metatarsals with their phalanges. The outer portion is formed by the calcaneus, the cuboid bone, the outer two metatarsals and the corresponding phalanges.

The inner portion of the arch, the instep, is high, only touching the ground at the calcaneus behind and at the lower end of the first metatarsal in front; the lower end of the first metatarsal is called the ball of the foot. The outer portion of the arch is low and rests on the ground.

The talus is the keystone of the arch and receives the body weight which it transmits through the pillars of the arch to the ground.

The longitudinal arch is supported chiefly by the long muscles of the leg and the short muscles of the foot; it is strengthened also by ligaments.

If it becomes flattened owing to muscular weakness, the foot is deprived of its normal spring and a shuffling, flat-footed gait develops.

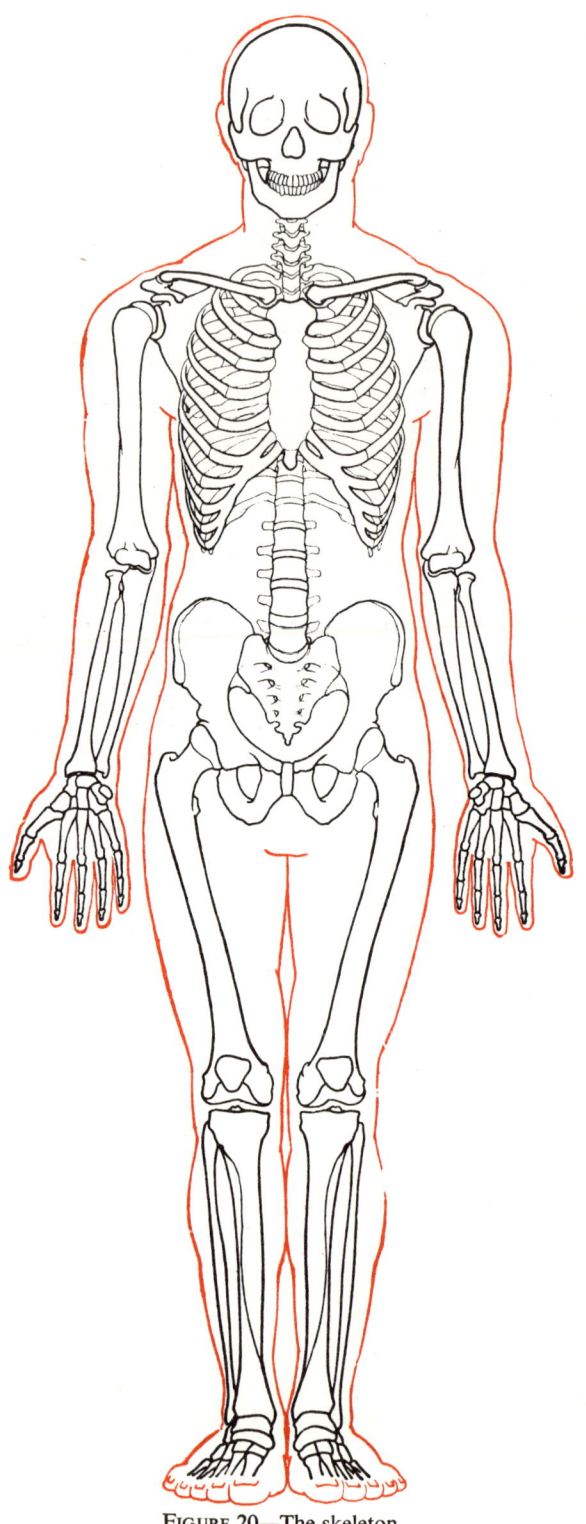
FIGURE 20—The skeleton

(2) The Transverse Arches

The tarsal and metatarsal bones are arranged with a slight convex, transverse curve on the upper surface of the foot and a slight concave, transverse curve on the sole of the foot. This arrangement forms a series of arches from one side of the foot to the other, extending from the lower ends of the metatarsals in front to the navicular and cuboid bones behind.

The transverse arches are supported by small muscles of the foot and by ligaments.

SECTION 2—JOINTS

A KNOWLEDGE of joints and their general structure, purpose and type and the direction of movement which they allow is of the greatest assistance in the understanding of muscle action.

A joint, or articulation, is formed by the meeting of two or more bones of the skeleton; it can allow free movement, slight movement or no movement at all, according to its type.

The joints of the body may be classified as follows:

(1) the *immovable* joint (Figure 21): this is a joint where the bones are united either by cartilage, for example, the cartilaginous junction between the first rib and sternum, or by a system of dovetailed edges as in the roof of the skull.

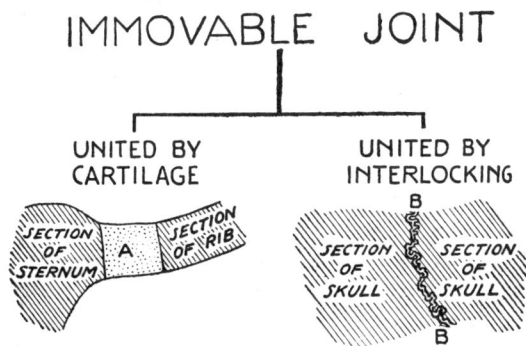

FIGURE 21—Immovable joints (diagrammatic)
A—Costal cartilage
B—Joint between skull bones

(2) the *slightly movable* joint (Figure 22): this consists of two bony surfaces united either by ligaments alone, such as the joint between the lower end of the tibia and fibula, or by ligaments with fibrous cartilage interposed between the bony surfaces, for example, the joints between the bodies of the vertebrae.

SLIGHTLY MOVABLE JOINT

UNITED BY LIGAMENTS ALONE

UNITED BY LIGAMENTS & FIBROUS CARTILAGE

FIGURE 22—Slightly movable joints (diagrammatic)
A—Ligament between lower end of tibia and fibula
B—Ligament between vertebrae
C—Cartilage

FREELY MOVABLE JOINT

GLIDING JOINT — HINGE JOINT — PIVOT JOINT — CONDYLOID JOINT — SADDLE JOINT — BALL & SOCKET JOINT

E   F   G   H   J   K

FIGURE 23—Freely movable joints (diagrammatic)
A—Cartilage   C—Synovial membrane
B—Capsule surrounding joint   D—Ligament

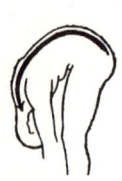 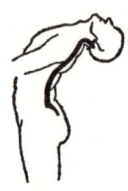 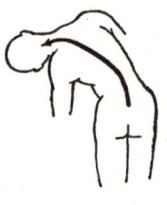 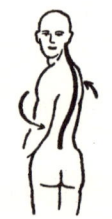

FLEXION   EXTENSION   LATERAL FLEXION   ROTATION

FIGURE 24—Movements of the vertebral column

(3) the *freely movable* joint (Figure 23): the two bone ends are covered with cartilage and connected by a fibrous capsule. The capsule is lined with smooth tissue called *synovial* membrane, which secretes a fluid to lubricate the joint, and is strengthened by ligaments, which are attached to the adjacent joint margins and whose number, strength and position depend on the particular function of the joint. A joint with a wide range of movement, such as the shoulder joint, has fewer ligaments than the hip joint which is less mobile, but which is adapted to bearing the body weight.

There are six types of freely movable joints which are illustrated in Figure 23 and may be described as follows.

(i) The *gliding* joint (E): flat surfaces are in contact. Examples are the joints between the articular processes of adjacent vertebrae and between the bones of the tarsus.

(ii) The *hinge* joint (F): such a joint allows movement in one plane only, at right angles to its transverse axis. Examples are the elbow, knee and ankle joints, and the joints of the fingers and toes.

(iii) The *pivot* joint (G): here a pivot-like process, held within a fibrous ring, rotates about its long axis. An example is the joint between the upper ends of the radius and ulna and another is that between the atlas and the vertical process of the axis.

(iv) The *condyloid* joint (H): this type of joint is one in which a convex, elliptical articular surface fits into a concave articular surface. The wrist joint is an example; it allows movements in all directions, but not rotation round its central axis.

(v) The *saddle* joint (J): the surfaces of such a joint are concavo-convex and the movements permitted are like those at a condyloid joint. The carpo-metacarpal joint of the thumb is an example.

(vi) The *ball and socket* joint (K): here a spherical head fits into a cup-like cavity. Movement is permitted in any direction as well as rotation round the central axis. The hip and shoulder joints are both of the ball and socket type.

The Joints of the Vertebral Column

The vertebral joints are:

(1) the slightly movable joints between the bodies of the vertebrae; these joints are maintained in position by two strong ligaments which run the whole length of the spine; one is attached firmly to the fronts of the vertebral bodies, and the other to the backs. Smaller ligaments bind together the adjacent surfaces of the bodies and intervertebral discs;

(2) the freely movable gliding joints between the articular surfaces projecting from the vertebral arches; each permits a gliding movement, the extent and direction of which depends upon its position in the vertebral column. The cervical and lumber vertebrae are more freely movable than the dorsal. In addition, each dorsal vertebra has four freely movable gliding joints for the corresponding ribs.

The space between the spinous processes and arches of adjacent vertebrae is filled by a special type of very powerful ligament which is yellow in colour and, unlike the normal type of ligament, is very elastic; if this ligament were not elastic, forward movement of the spine would be impossible.

The movements of the vertebral column (Figure 24) are:

(1) movement forward or *flexion*; this is the most extensive of all the movements and is freest in the lumbar region;

(2) movement backward or *extension*; this movement is freest in the cervical region;

(3) movement sideways or *lateral flexion*; this movement may take place

at any part of the column, but is freest in the cervical and lumbar regions;

(4) *rotation*; this occurs to a slight extent in the cervical region, is freer in the upper dorsal region, and gradually diminishes in the lower dorsal region; it is absent in the lumbar region.

Movements in the dorsal region are limited in order to reduce interference with respiration to a minimum.

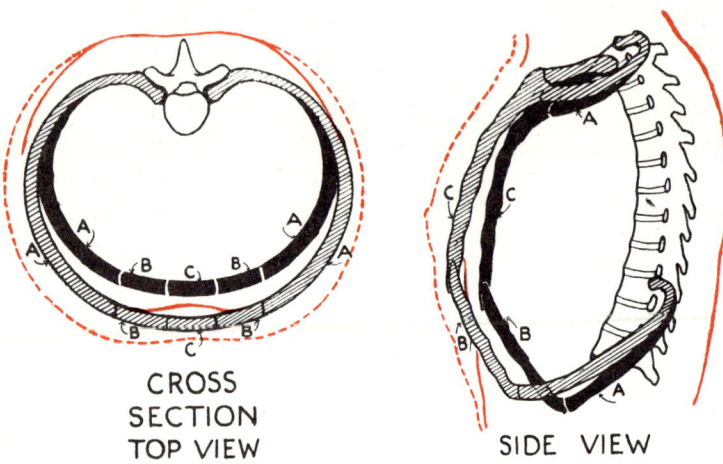

FIGURE 25—Diagram of the movements of the thorax in breathing
(Shaded outline shows inspiration; dark outline indicates expiration)
A—Rib
B—Costal cartilage
C—Sternum

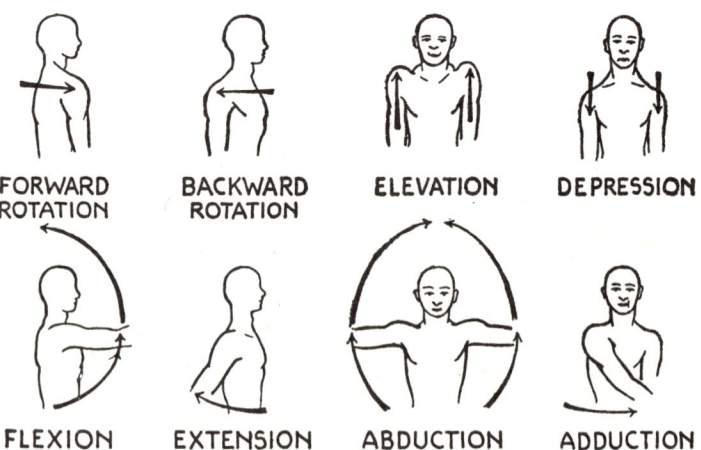

FIGURE 26—The movements of the upper limb

The Rib Joints

The head and neck of each rib form two freely movable gliding joints with the body and transverse process of the corresponding dorsal vertebrae. Each rib has its own range and variety of movement, but the movements of all are combined in breathing.

Breathing in, or *inspiration*, enlarges the circumference of the thorax; breathing out, or *expiration*, decreases the circumference (Figure 25).

Inspiration is a combined movement of the ribs, costal cartilages and sternum; the direction of movement of the front and sides of the chest wall is upward, forward and outward; on expiration, movement in the reverse direction takes place. These movements may be more clearly understood by reference to Figure 25, in which the outward movement of the bodies of the ribs and sternum and the forward movement of the costal cartilage are shown; in the side view it can be seen that the sternum, costal cartilage and ribs also move slightly upward. The combined movement performed by the ribs and sternum during inspiration can be demonstrated as follows: clasp the hands in front of the body, the hands representing the sternum and the bent elbows, the ribs; then move the hands upward and slightly forward and at the same time the elbows outward and upward.

The movement of an individual rib may be compared to that of the handle of a bucket, except that the extremities of a rib do not remain level with one another during inspiration and expiration.

Joints of the Shoulder Girdle

The joint between the sternum and clavicle is a freely movable gliding joint; it is the only point at which the shoulder girdle articulates with the trunk. This joint permits movement of the clavicle in all directions.

The outer end of the clavicle forms the *acromioclavicular* joint with the acromion process of the scapula; this is a freely movable joint and permits gliding movements.

Both the above joints are subjected to considerable strains and are therefore supported by strong ligaments.

The Shoulder Joint

The shoulder joint is of the ball and socket type formed by the hemispherical head of the humerus and the shallow glenoid fossa of the scapula. Structurally it is a weak joint and for such strength as it does possess, it is dependent more upon the muscles which surround it than on the ligaments.

The articular cavity, or *glenoid fossa*, which receives the head of the humerus is deepened by the attachment of a ring of fibrous cartilage round its rim.

The whole joint is enveloped in a capsule and is strengthened by certain ligaments above and in front; seven important muscles give their support mainly to the upper part of the joint capsule. The lower aspect of the capsule is thus the least protected part, so when a dislocation of the shoulder occurs, it is usually through this lower and weaker part of the capsule.

The movements of the upper limb (Figure 26) can be described as follows.
   (1) Movements of the shoulder girdle:
      (i) forward or *forward rotation*;
      (ii) bracing the shoulders backward or *backward rotation*;
      (iii) shrugging the shoulders or *elevation*;
      (iv) downward movement of the shoulders or *depression*.
   (2) Movements of the shoulder joint:
      (i) forward elevation of the upper arm or *flexion*;
      (ii) backward swinging of the upper arm or *extension*;
      (iii) sideways movement of the upper arm away from the body or *abduction*,
      (iv) movement of the upper arm from the abducted position towards the body and across the chest towards the opposite shoulder; this is called *adduction*;

(v) outward rotation of the upper arm or *external rotation*; the extent of this movement can be measured in two ways; if the arm is held as in Figure 27, position A—the elbow bent to a right angle—and the forearm is then raised in a backward direction, position B, the amount of external rotation present can be gauged; the same movement occurs, when with the elbow at the side and bent at a right angle, position C, the forearm is carried outwards away from the midline, position D;

(vi) the reverse movement, called *internal rotation*; this may be demonstrated by moving the forearm downward and backward from position A to position E.

Internal rotation also occurs when the forearm is placed across the small of the back. It must be borne in mind that both external and internal rotation are purely shoulder movements; no rotation whatsoever occurs at the elbow, though it might appear so at first sight;

(vii) circular movement or *circumduction*; this can combine all the above movements.

The Elbow Joint (Figure 28)

The elbow joint is of the hinge type and is formed by the articulation of the lower end of the humerus, the upper extremity of the ulna and the head of the radius.* The elbow joint is strengthened by two strong ligaments on each side and by powerful muscles in front and behind.

The movements at the elbow joint are:

(1) bending the elbow or *flexion*;

(2) straightening the elbow or *extension*.

*The head of the radius increases the stability of this hinge joint, but is not absolutely essential to its function. When fractured, it is often removed and the functional result is usually very good.

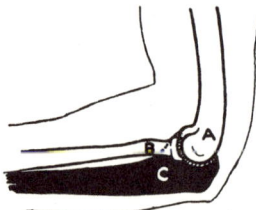

FIGURE 28—Left elbow joint
A—Lower end of humerus
B—Upper end of radius
C—Upper end of ulna

The Joints between the Radius and Ulna (Figure 29)

The upper and lower articulation between the radius and the ulna are both pivot joints; in the upper joint the neck of the radius rotates within a ring shaped ligament, and in the lower joint the end of the radius revolves round the ulna.

The movements in which the radius and ulna take part are:

(1) turning the palm of the hand downward towards the ground or *pronation*; after this movement the radius lies across the ulna;

(2) turning the palm upward or *supination*; this is the reverse movement; after full supination the radius lies to the outer side of and parallel to the ulna.

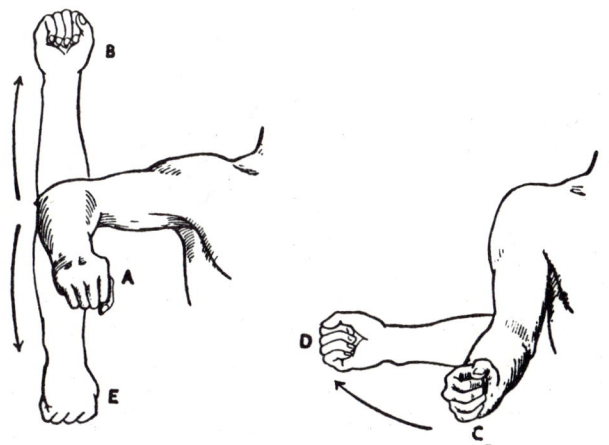

FIGURE 27—External and internal rotation of the upper arm
    A—Mid-position   D—Full external rotation
    B—Full external rotation   E—Full internal rotation
    C—Mid-position

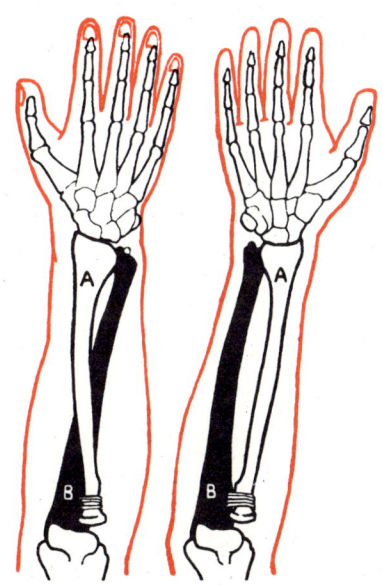

PRONATION   SUPINATION

FIGURE 29—The joints between the radius and the ulna
(Right forearm)
    A—Radius   B—Ulna

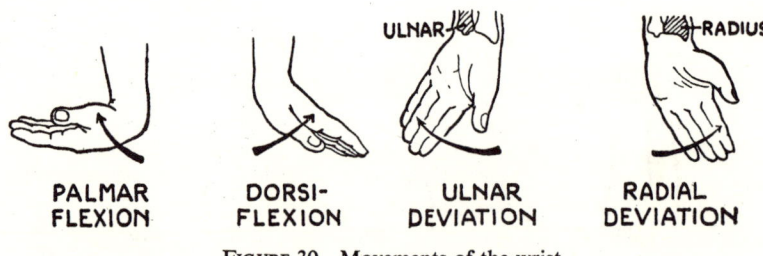

FIGURE 30—Movements of the wrist

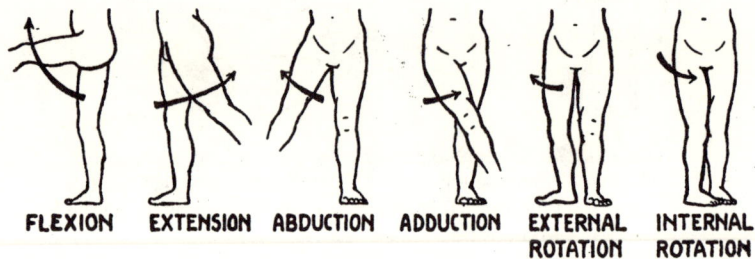

FIGURE 31—Movements of the hip joint

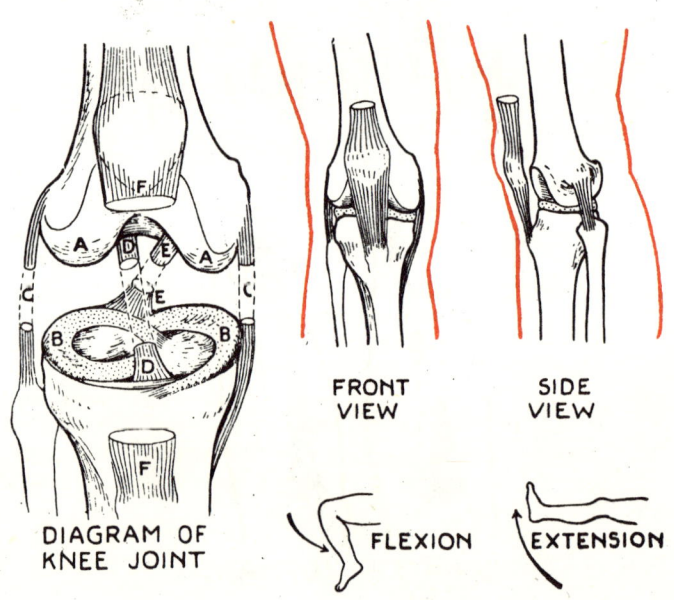

FIGURE 32—The knee joint (diagrammatic)
A—Condyle of femur
B—Cartilage
C—Internal and external ligaments
D—Anterior cruciate ligament
E—Posterior cruciate ligament
F—Quadriceps tendon

The Wrist Joint

The wrist joint is a condyloid articulation formed by the lower end of the radius, a disc of cartilage attached to the lower extremity of the ulna, and the upper aspect of the carpus. It is strengthened by ligaments on both sides and at the back and front of the joint.

The movements permitted at the wrist joint (Figure 30) are:

(1) forward bending or *palmar flexion*;

(2) backward bending or *dorsiflexion*;

(3) sideways movement; when the ulnar border of the hand is moved in such a way that it decreases the angle between itself and the ulna, the movement is called *ulnar deviation*; the opposite movement, that is, moving the radial border of the hand, is called *radial deviation*;

(4) circular movement, or *circumduction*, is a combination of all the above movements.

Any force which may be transmitted through the wrist joint is first taken by the lower end of the radius; it is in this part of the bone that a fracture so commonly occurs as a result of a backfire injury when cranking a car or as a result of a fall; it is called a *Colles* fracture.

The Hip Joint

The hip joint is a ball and socket articulation formed by the cup-shaped cavity of the acetabulum and the head of the femur. It is surrounded by a strong capsule and very strong ligaments upon which it is largely dependent for its stability; the ligaments in front of the hip joint are the strongest in the body.

Movements of the hip joint (Figure 31) are:

(1) raising the thigh or *flexion*;

(2) bracing the thigh backward or *extension*;

(3) raising the thigh sideways away from the other leg or *abduction*;

(4) moving the thigh from a position of abduction across the other leg, called *adduction*;

(5) rotation of the thigh outward or *external rotation*;

(6) rotation of the thigh inward or *internal rotation*;

(7) circular movement or *circumduction*; this is a combination of the above movements.

Dislocation of the normal hip joint occurs when very considerable violence is applied. It often results from a severe impact against the knees when a person is in the sitting position, which drives the head of the femur backward over the margin of the acetabulum. It occurs in motor accidents when the knees are impacted violently against the dash board.

The Knee Joint (Figure 32)

The knee joint is made up of the two condyles of the femur and the upper end of the tibia; it is a hinge joint. Two crescent shaped pieces of cartilage are attached to the upper end of the tibia; the purpose of these cartilages is to provide a smooth and accurately fitting articulation btween the surfaces of the condyles and the upper end of the tibia.

The knee joint has a loose capsule supported by a strong ligament on both sides. There are also two strong ligaments called *cruciate* ligaments, which arise from the tibia and are attached between the condyles of the femur; these ligaments are directed diagonally across the middle of the joint, in such a way that they do not interfere with joint movement, but prevent the femur slipping forward or backward on the tibia. The front of the knee joint is supported by the very strong combined tendon of the muscle which extends the knee, called the *quadriceps*. The patella, which is fixed within this tendon, articulates with the groove between the two condyles.

The knee joint appears to be one of the least secure joints, because the leverage imposed upon it by the two longest bones in the body is very great, the joint surfaces are not close fitting and the movement allowed is considerable; nevertheless this joint is very strong owing to the support of the powerful ligaments and muscles around it. Dislocation only occurs as a result of extreme violence.

The condition of 'water on the knee,' or *synovitis*, is caused by an excessive secretion of synovial fluid as a result of disease or injury to the joint. Synovitis can occur within any joint which has a synovial membrane, that is to say within any freely movable type of joint. It is seen more commonly in the knee than elsewhere because this joint is not only very exposed to minor strains and injuries, but it also has a relatively large and superficial synovial membrane which makes the detection of fluid a simple matter.

The cartilages in the knee are often damaged; they may then interfere with the normal working of the joint. Injury to a cartilage may be caused by a violent twisting movement of the body when one foot is firmly fixed on the ground with the knee bent; if, for example, the individual has all his weight upon the right foot with his knee bent and he twists suddenly in an anti-clockwise direction, he may injure his inner cartilage; if he twists in a clockwise direction the outer cartilage may be damaged.

Immediately after a cartilage has been injured the knee joint may remain locked; in such a case any would-be helpers should resist the temptation to unlock the joint. Medical assistance should be obtained if possible, for it is a great help to the doctor in forming an exact diagnosis if he sees the joint in the locked position; he is then able to furnish an accurate report to the surgeon.

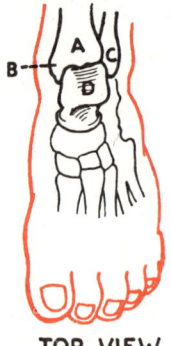
TOP VIEW

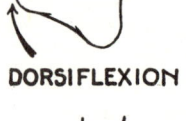
DORSIFLEXION

PLANTAR FLEXION

FIGURE 33—The anatomy and movements of the ankle joint
A—Lower end of tibia   C—Lower end of fibula (external malleolus)
B—Internal malleolus   D—Upper articular surface of talus

The Ankle Joint (Figure 33)

The ankle joint is formed by the lower end of the tibia with its malleolus, the lower end of the fibula, and the upper articular surface of the talus.

It is a hinge joint and its capsule is supported by strong ligaments on both sides with smaller ligaments at the front and back. The ligaments at the side are sometimes ruptured when the ankle is twisted, but quite often the ligaments remain intact, tearing off a piece of bone from the lower end of the fibula or from the internal malleolus.

Movements of the ankle joint (Figure 33) are:
(1) raising the foot upward towards the knee or *dorsiflexion*;
(2) bending the foot downward away from the knee or *plantar flexion*.

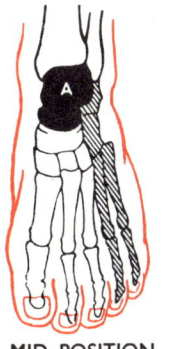 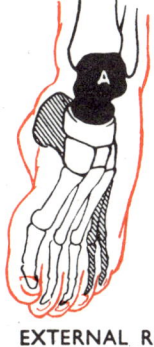

FIGURE 34—Inversion of the left foot
A—Talus

MID POSITION
B

EXTERNAL ROTATION
C

The Joints between the Talus and Calcaneus and between the Talus and Navicular (Figure 34)

These are strongly made gliding joints; they are important in so far as they permit turning of the sole of the foot to face inward and outward called *inversion* and *eversion* respectively. The range of eversion is very small.

In Figure 34 it will be seen that the talus remains still while the foot moves round it from position B to position C. These joints also permit a limited movement of the forepart of the foot inward, or *internal rotation*, and outward, *external rotation*. It is important to understand that no inversion, eversion or rotation can occur at the ankle joint; movements there are purely dorsiflexion and plantar flexion.

Comparison of Function of the Upper and Lower Limbs

The functions and movements of the upper limb differ widely from those of the lower limb, although there is much similarity of anatomical structure between the limbs themselves. The reason for this can be explained on a purely mechanical basis.

Vertebrate life on this planet was represented by primitive creatures, like lizards, when the terrestrial stage of evolution had been reached; all four limbs were then used for propulsion only, the body weight being supported on the belly wall. During ensuing stages, certain of these primitive vertebrates began to use their limbs as a means of support as well as progression, and their abdomens were raised off the ground. This development gave them big advantages; they were more agile in acquiring food and escaping from their enemies. Many of those vertebrates which did not undergo this change failed to survive, but one or two representatives still exist today for example,, the crocodile, which lives in the protective environment of rivers. On the other hand some vertebrates went a stage further than that of lifting their bellies off the ground, and began to reach up for their food and balance on the hind limbs; at this stage the higher vertebrates, man and the apes, began to evolve, and man soon gained an advantage over the apes, because he adapted himself to the fully erect posture; this gave him an increased field of vision which helped him procure food more easily and keep a keener watch for enemies.

The abdominal musculature became further developed to support the abdominal contents and to maintain the body in the upright position; the muscles which extend the spine, hip and knee, became especially powerful. The fore limbs became more mobile and generally lighter in structure, and the hind limbs became stronger and in certain respects less mobile. Mobility and precision of movement of the upper limb were gained at the expense of muscle power and joint stability; the reverse process took place in the lower limb. The wrist and ankle joints, for example, have now reached a stage in evolution where they have very little similarity in function or movement;

the former has become adapted in structure to allow free mobility of the carpus, enabling the fingers to perform fine and accurate movements, whereas the latter has become adapted to serve the special function of weight bearing and allows only such movements to occur as are necessary for the propulsion of the body. The ankle joint would be quite unstable for weight-bearing and locomotion if it permitted more movement than dorsiflexion and plantar flexion.

The movements of the tarsus, namely inversion, eversion and rotation, have been developed to enable man to walk on uneven surfaces. The stability of the foot as a lever for progression is not in any way impaired by such movements, because its width and the close proximity to the ground of the joints at which these movements occur, counteract any tendency of the foot to turn over accidentally under normal conditions of exercise.

SECTION 3—THE MUSCULAR SYSTEM

The muscles of the human body constitute about 45 per cent of its total weight. There are three varieties of muscle tissue:

(1) that which produces movements of the bony skeleton, under voluntary control, called *striped* or *voluntary* muscle;

(2) that which forms the muscular coats of the intestine, bladder, arteries and many other structures; it is not under voluntary control and is known as *unstriped* or *involuntary* muscle; (this fortunately does not mean that the action of the bowels and bladder are involuntary—the reasons for this will be discussed in Chapter II);

(3) that which is striped but involuntary; this kind of muscle is found only in the heart and is called *cardiac* muscle.

This book is concerned with the first variety of muscle tissue only.

The Structure of Muscle

Voluntary muscle is made up of a large number of fibres. A muscle fibre is approximately one and a half inches long and about as thick as a human hair; under the microscope it has a characteristic transverse striping which is not present in involuntary muscle. Each fibre is enclosed in an elastic sheath and is attached to other fibres to form longitudinal strands, which are arranged in parallel bundles. The fleshy belly of a muscle is composed of an enormous number of these bundles.

Muscle Tendon (Figure 35)

The extremities of each muscle are attached to bony or other structures either by bands of strong white fibrous tissue called *tendon* or by direct attachment of muscle fibres. In Figure 35, the muscle bundles can be seen converging towards the tendon. As a general rule, the end of the muscle nearer the trunk is attached either by its muscle fibres or by a short tendon, whereas the end further away from the trunk is more often attached by a tendon which is of greater length.

Tendons make possible the concentration of the force of powerful muscles on small areas; the muscles which extend the knee, for example, concentrate their pull by this means on a small projection of bone in front of the upper end of the tibia or shin bone. Tendons also enable muscles to act from a distance, for example, the long tendons of the muscles of the forearm which bend the fingers; the mass of muscle is thus closer to the source of its blood supply and away from the fingers whose mobility it would hinder.

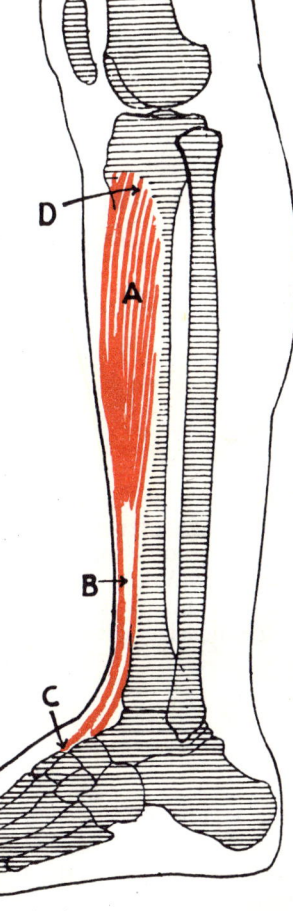

FIGURE 35—Muscles of the leg showing muscle bundles merging into a tendon
A—Muscle bundles   C—Insertion
B—Tendon   D—Origin

The Origin and Insertion of Muscle

The main function of voluntary muscle is to produce and control movements of the body and to maintain natural posture by acting upon the bony structure. An individual muscle is usually attached by a tendon to the bone it moves: this point of attachment is called the *insertion* (Figure 35); the muscle is fixed at its other end either with or without a tendon to another bone or to some other structure; this point of attachment is called the *origin* (Figure 35). Not all muscles have these simple origins and insertions on account of variations in shape, size and location.

The Reverse Action of Muscle

The simplest mechanical form of muscle action is contraction, by which the points of origin and insertion are drawn towards each other; muscles can therefore work in a reverse way, if the bone which is usually moved, is fixed; a simple example illustrates this fact; in opening a door, the door is pulled by the moving arm towards the body, but if the door is locked and the attempt to open it is continued, the hand and arm remain fixed and the body is pulled towards the door.

Lever Action of Muscle

Muscles are arranged in the body in such a way as to concentrate the maximum power in the minimum space; this economy of effort is mainly brought about by a system of levers and pulleys.

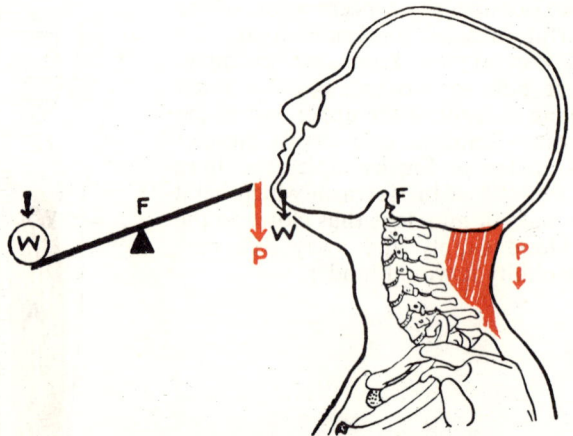

FIGURE 36—First type of lever and
its action at the joint between the skull and atlas

There are three different types of lever action employed in the body. Figure 36 shows a diagrammatic example of the first type; the fulcrum F is between the weight W and the power P. In the body, F is the joint between the atlas and the skull, W is the weight of the skull and P is the power, or pull, exerted by the muscles which draw the head backward.

In Figure 37, showing the second type, W is between F and P; the action of the calf muscles raising the body on the toes illustrate this in the body.

The calf muscles are working at a mechanical advantage, for if we multiply the weight by its distance from the fulcrum, the product is equal to the power multiplied by the distance of its point of application from the fulcrum; hence, assuming the distance of P to F and W to F is in the ratio of 3 : 2, a man weighing 150 pounds would require to exert a pull of only 100 pounds in his calf muscles to lift himself on his toes.

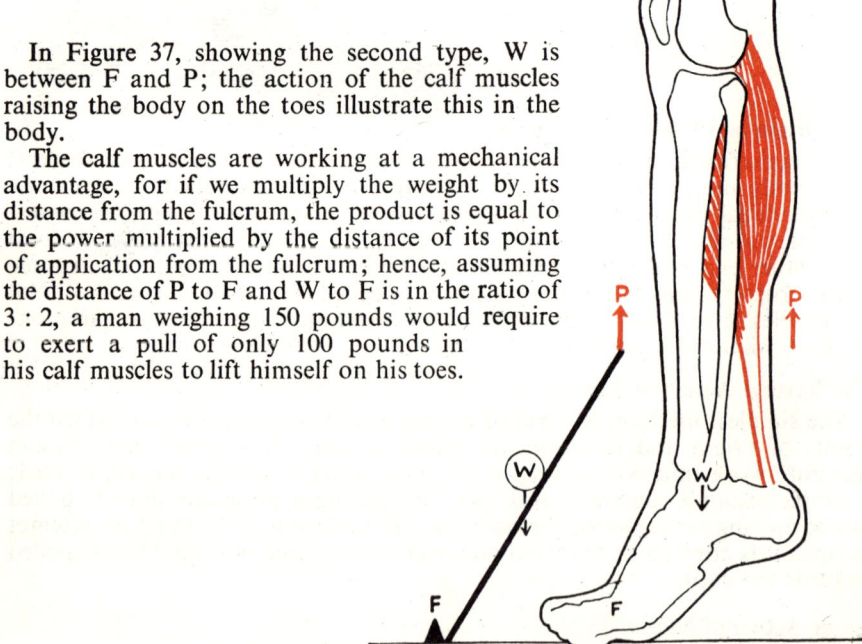

FIGURE 37—Second type of lever and
its action at the ankle joint

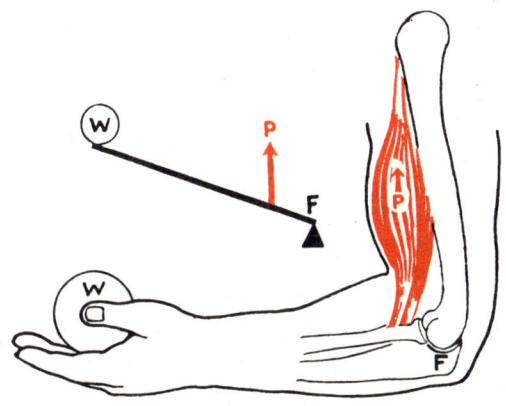

FIGURE 38—Third type of lever and its action at the elbow joint

Figure 38, showing the third type of lever, demonstrates that muscles working in this way are at a mechanical disadvantage for P is between F and W.

This form of leverage is employed when the elbow is flexed. It is the type used most frequently in the body. If we assume that the distance from W to F is about 7 times greater than the distance from P to F, the muscles which flex the elbow must exert a pull of $7 \times 5 = 35$ pounds in order to lift a five pound weight held in the hand.

Pulley action is employed in the body to change the direction of muscular effort; friction at the pulley is minimised by the use of double layered ensheathing membranes or of small sacs containing a lubricating fluid, interposed between the tendon and the point of maximum pressure. For example, the tendons of the muscles which bend the fingers move backwards and forwards beneath the fibrous tunnels, which bind them closely to the bones of the fingers; if the tendon were not covered by a sheath containing lubricating fluid, there would be much friction between the tendon and overlying structures.

Small disc-shaped bones, called *sesamoid bones*, are sometimes incorporated in the tendon as it glides round a bony prominence; they are usually between one-eighth and a quarter of an inch in diameter, but the patella, described in Chapter I, is also a sesamoid bone. The purpose of sesamoid bones is to improve leverage by preventing friction and by changing the direction of the force of pull.

Muscles Acting upon more than One Joint

There are many instances in the body where a muscle acts upon more than one joint. A muscle can produce the same type of movement, for example, flexion in each of the joints over which it passes or it may produce flexion in one joint and extension in another; the two different types of movement may be produced simultaneously or separately. For example, the long tendons which flex the fingers pass over several joints, producing in each one the same type of movement, namely flexion; the quadriceps muscle, however, a part of which originates from the front of the hip bone, can flex the hip and extend the knee; in walking or running, it is performing both movements; when the knee joint is held fixed, it flexes the hip; if the hip joint is fixed, it extends the knee.

Types of Muscular Work

It has already been mentioned that the simplest form of muscle action is contraction by which the points of origin and insertion are drawn towards each other. This type of muscle work is sometimes called *concentric*; for example, when picking up a book from a table, the muscles which flex the elbow are doing concentric work.

Static work is done when the muscles do not shorten or lengthen visibly—the book is held steady in the hand. The muscles of posture perform static work when a person is standing still.

Eccentric work is done when muscles extend and give in to resistance; when the book is replaced on the table, the muscles which flex the elbow, extend as the book is lowered on to the table.

THE INDIVIDUAL MUSCLES

There are 215 pairs of muscles in the body; of these the most important will be described in detail, and some of the less important will be briefly mentioned. It must be understood that in dealing with the muscles of the trunk, the description refers only to the muscles of one side, unless otherwise stated.

MUSCLES OF THE TRUNK

1. Muscles of the Neck

(i) The *sternomastoid* (Figure 39): each muscle passes obliquely across the side of the neck.

Origin: from the upper part of the sternum and the inner third of the clavicle.

Insertion: into the mastoid process of the skull behind the ear.

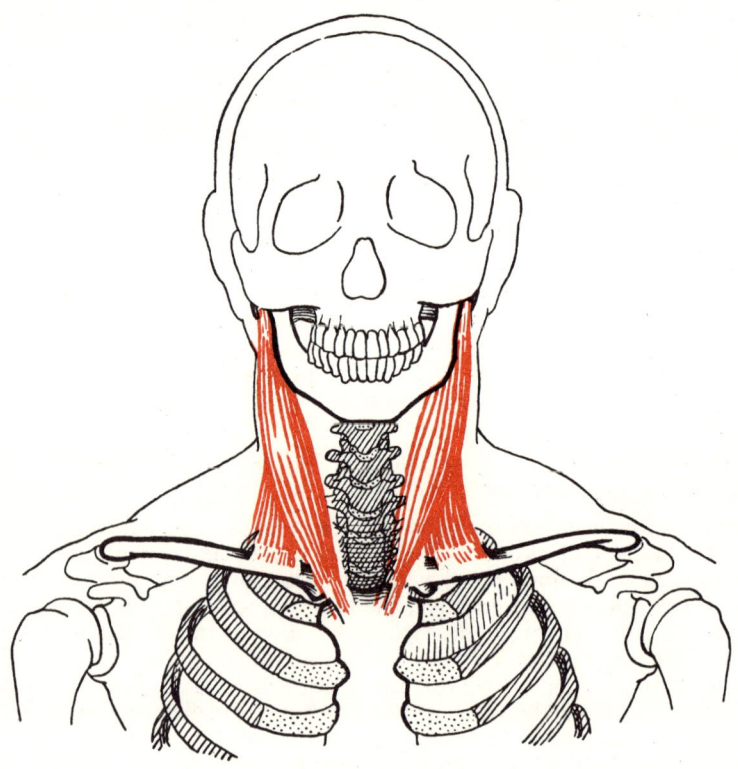

FIGURE 39—The sternomastoids

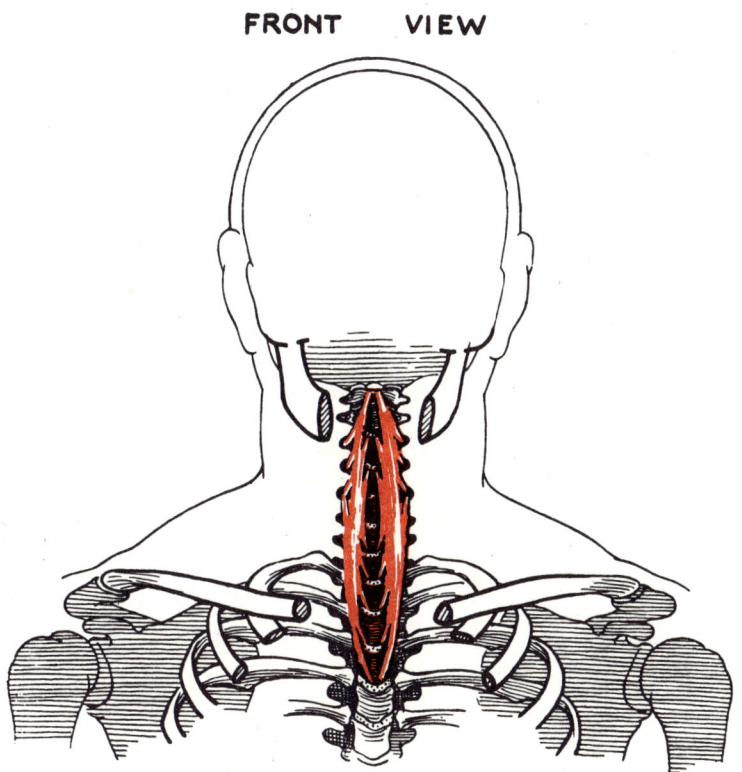

FIGURE 40—The longi colli
(Part of the ribs, sternum, clavicles and jaw
bone have been cut away)

Action: contraction of the muscle of one side draws the head towards the shoulder of the same side; it also rotates the head to face towards the opposite shoulder. Both muscles acting together with the sternum as the fixed point, flex the head and the cervical part of the vertebral column; but if the head is fixed by other muscular contraction, the sternomastoids are capable of acting as accessory muscles of respiration by helping to elevate the thorax.

The deformity known as *wryneck* is due to a chronically contracted sternomastoid; there is another condition in which the sternomastoids are affected, called *spasmodic torticollis*. Sufferers from it are unable to keep their heads still, either jerking them quickly or turning them in a slow and sustained fashion. It is due to a nervous disorder and other muscles of the neck and head are often affected.

(ii) The *longus colli* (long muscle of the neck, Figure 40): each muscle is situated on the anterior surface of the vertebral column between the atlas and the third dorsal vertebra.

Origin: from the fronts of the lower cervical and upper three dorsal vertebrae.

Insertion: into the fronts of the upper cervical vertebrae.

Action: its chief action is to flex the cervical portion of the vertebral column.

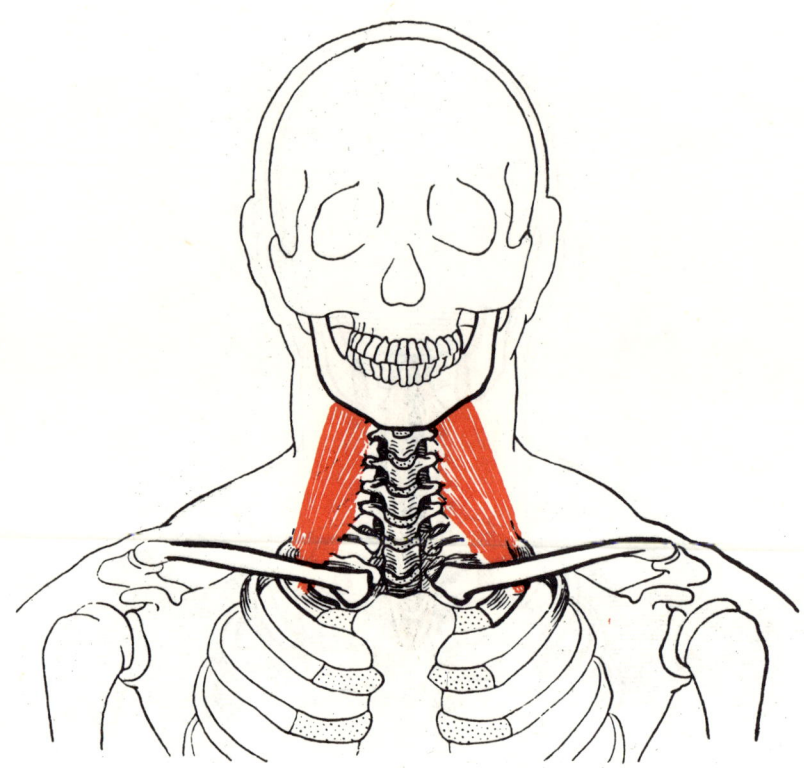

FIGURE 41—The scaleni

(iii) The *scaleni* (scalene muscles,* Figure 41): there are three of these muscles on each side of the neck beneath the sternomastoids.

Origins: from the transverse processes of the cervical vertebrae.

Insertions: two into the upper surface of the body of the first rib and the third into the body of the second rib.

Actions: the scaleni bend the neck forward when acting together; when those of one side only are acting, they bend the neck to that side and turn the face toward the opposite shoulder. They can act as accessory muscles of respiration like the sternomastoid; the runner in a quarter-mile race usually finishes with his head and neck thrown well back in order to make full use of these accessory muscles of respiration.

*Scalene means with sides of differing lengths.

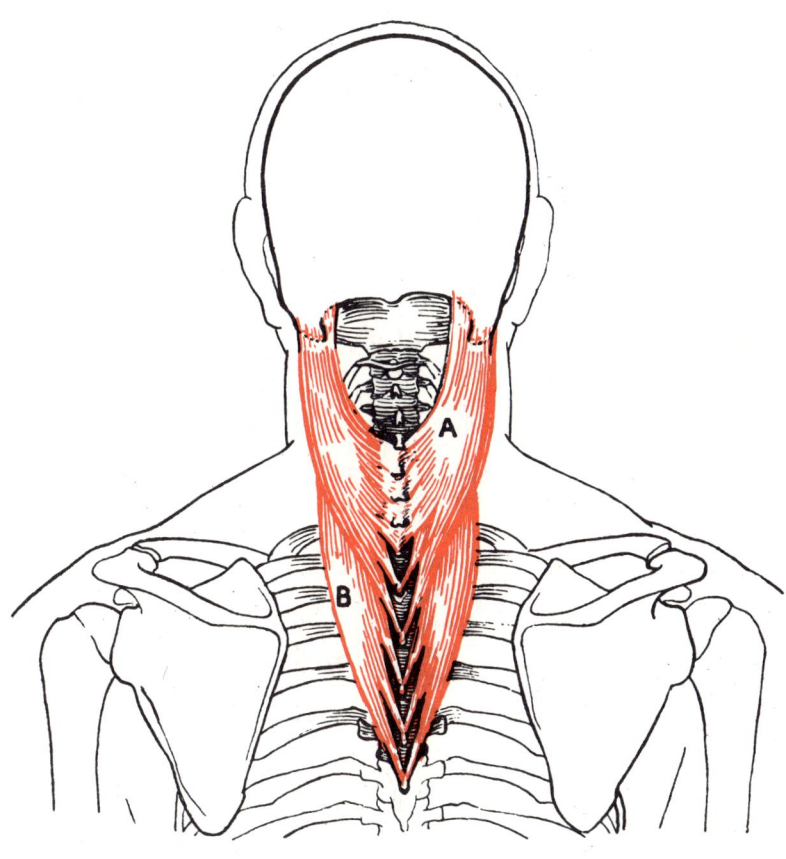

FIGURE 42
A—Splenius capitis   B—Splenius cervicis

(iv) The *splenius capitis* (the splint of the head, Figure 42): this muscle is situated over the posterior aspect of the cervical and upper four dorsal vertebrae. It takes origin from the spinous processes of cervical and dorsal vertebrae and is inserted into the mastoid process of the skull. Both muscles acting together draw the head directly backward; each splenius muscle acting separately bends the head to its own side.

(v) The *splenius cervicis* (the splint of the neck, Figure 42): arises from the spinous processes of the third to the sixth dorsal vertebrae and is inserted into the transverse processes of the upper two or three cervical vertebrae. It acts in conjunction with the splenius capitis.

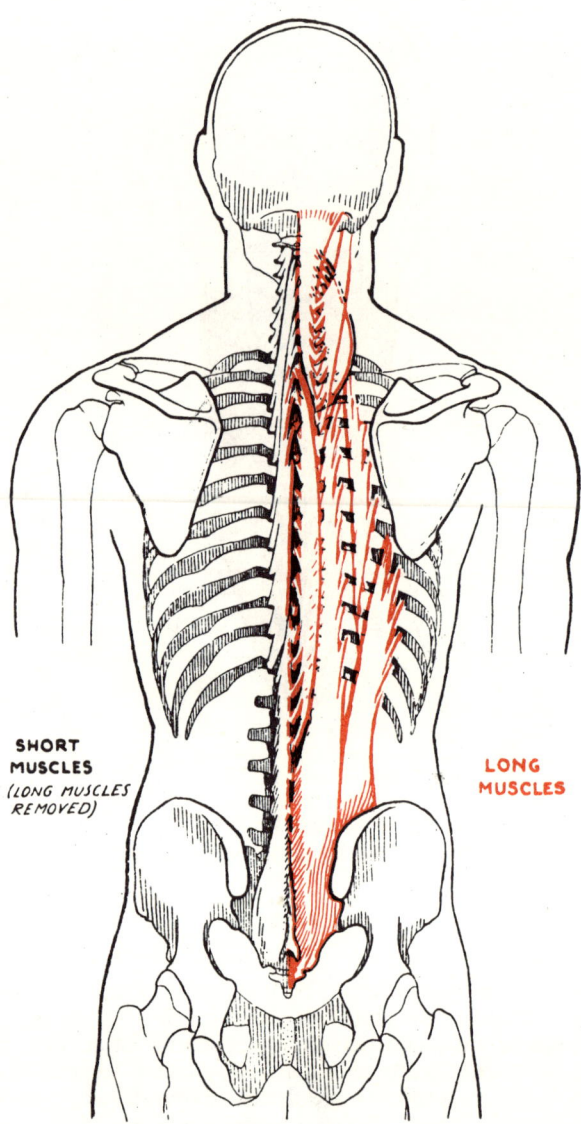

FIGURE 43—Attachments of long and short spinal muscles (diagrammatic)

2. Muscles of the Spine

The muscles of the spine may be divided into two main groups each consisting of many muscles.

(i) the *long*, for example the large *sacrospinalis* (muscle of the sacrum and spine) on each side of the lower part of the back;

(ii) the *short*, consisting of (*a*) muscles rotating one vertebra upon another, and (*b*) muscles extending or tilting one vertebra upon another.

The long spinal muscles (Figures 43 and 44) extend from the sacrum to the base of the skull and lie behind the angles of the ribs and the transverse processes of the vertebrae.

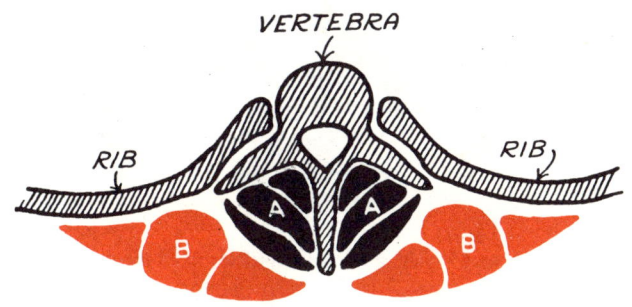

FIGURE 44—Arrangements of the short (A) and long muscles (B) of the spine, viewed in section (diagrammatic)

Origins: from the sacrum, the innominate bone, the spinous and transverse processes of the lumbar, dorsal and cervical vertebrae and the ligaments connecting these bones.

Insertions: into the spinous processes of the lumbar, dorsal and cervical vertebrae, the base of the skull and the angles of the ribs; the object of this arrangement is to distribute the pull of the long spinal muscles over the widest possible area and allow movements of extension at different levels of the sdine.

Actions: these muscles are mainly powerful extensors of the spine.

The *short* muscles of the spine (Figures 43 and 44) fill in the spaces between the spines of the vertebrae and their transverse processes and lie underneath the various divisions of the long muscles.

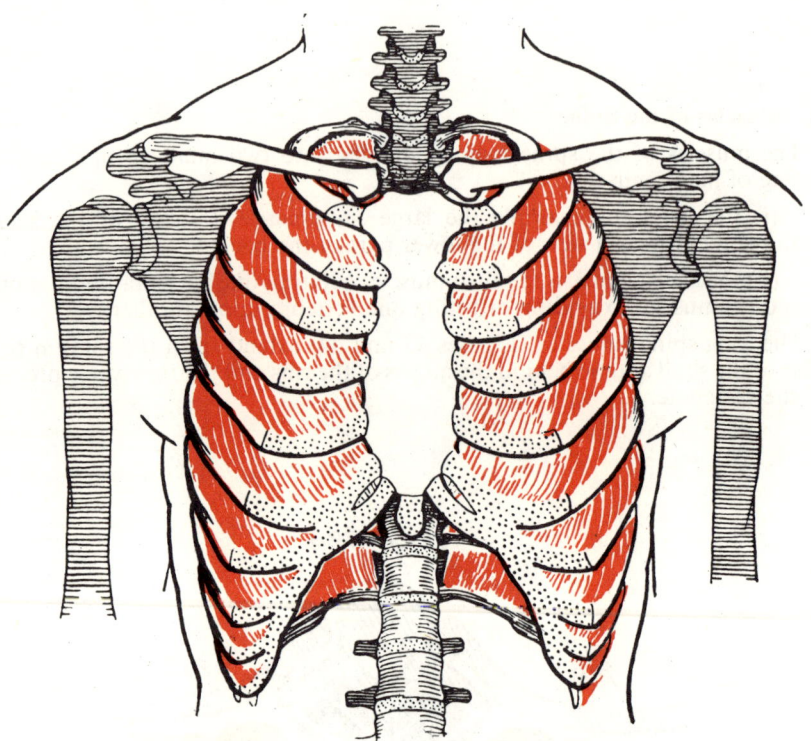

FIGURE 45—The intercostal muscles from the front

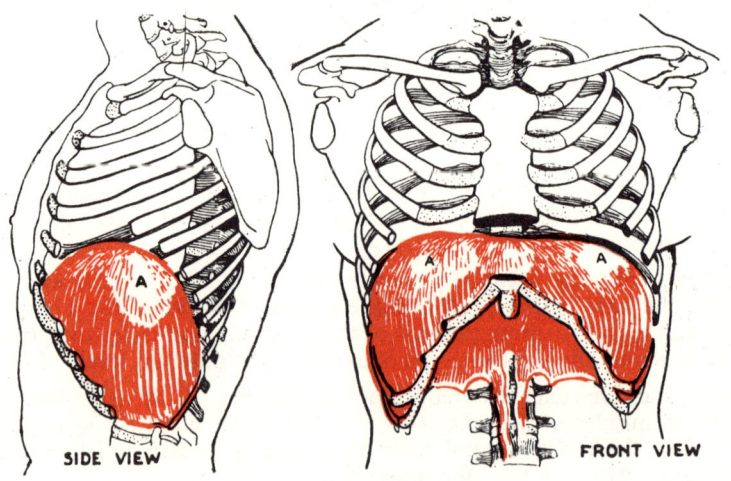

FIGURE 46—The diaphragm
A—Tendon
(The ribs and sternum have been partly removed)

3. Muscles of the Thorax

(i) The *intercostales* (muscles between ribs, Figure 45): these muscles, consisting of an internal and external layer, lie between the adjacent borders of the ribs; their main action is to pull the ribs together. There are several other small muscles which assist in moving the ribs.

(ii) The *diaphragm* or midriff (Figure 46): this is a dome-shaped muscle which separates the thoracic from the abdominal cavity. The middle portion of the dome is composed of a broad sheet of tendon, shaped like a three bladed leaf.

Origin: in front, from the lower end of the sternum and the costal cartilages of the lower six ribs on either side; behind, from the twelfth rib and the bodies and transverse processes of the upper lumbar vertebrae.

Insertion: all the fibres from these numerous origins converge to be inserted into the central tendon.

Action: the diaphragm is the principal muscle of respiration. In direct contact with the upper surface are the lungs and heart, and in contact with the lower, are the liver in the middle and on the right, and the stomach with other abdominal organs on the left.

The lower ribs become fixed in normal inspiration to enable the diaphragm to draw down the central tendon during its contraction. It moves downwards without much alteration in shape, expanding the lung above it and pushing the abdominal contents downwards. When the limit of downward movement is reached, which is decided by the resistance of the abdominal wall, the central tendon becomes the fixed point, being pressed hard against the abdominal contents; as a result the lower ribs move slightly forward, outward and upward thus increasing the diameter of the lower part of the chest. Normal expiration is mainly the result of the elastic recoil of the thoracic walls, helped by the contraction of the abdominal muscles which push the abdominal contents back into their previous position.

4. Muscles of the Abdomen

The anterior and lateral muscles of the abdominal wall consist of three pairs of broad sheet-like muscles, namely:

(i) the *external obliques*,
(ii) the *internal obliques*,
(iii) the *transverse muscles*, and
(iv) the long pillar-like *recti abdominis* or vertical muscles of the abdomen.

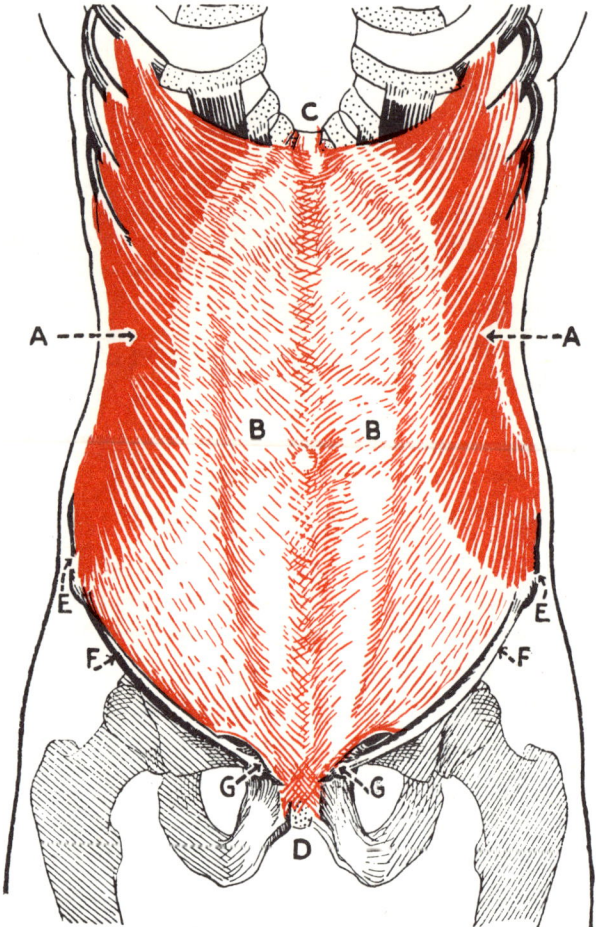

FIGURE 47—The external oblique muscles of the abdomen
A—Fibres of external oblique   B—Aponeurosis of external oblique extending over rectus
CD—Junction of aponeuroses in midline   E—Crest of ilium   F—Inguinal ligament
G—Crest of pubis

The origins, insertions and actions of these eight muscles are complex, and stress is here laid upon their functions rather than their precise actions.

The oblique and transverse muscles cover the abdomen in front and on each side, lying in close contact one with another; the two recti abdominis, one on each side of the midline, extend the whole length of the front of the abdomen.

The outer layer of the abdominal musculature is formed by the two *external oblique* muscles (Figure 47), each of which is a broad, flat muscle extending from the lower ribs to the groin, its fibres directed obliquely downward and inward.

The fleshy part of the muscle emerges into a thin but very broad, tendinous sheet called an *aponeurosis*, which transmits the pull of each muscle over a wide insertion.

Origin: from the lower eight ribs.

Insertion: by means of the aponeuroses of the two muscles which blend with one another in the midline of the body, represented by an imaginary line CD between the sternum and the pubic junction. Each aponeurosis is also inserted below into the *crest of the ilium** and into a strong ligament—the *inguinal ligament*—which is a condensation of the lower fibres of the aponeurosis of the external oblique, and stretches between its attachments to the crest of the ilium and fibres of the crest of the pubis.†

*The crest of the ilium is the uppermost margin of the innominate bone.
†A ridge of bone each side of the junction of the two pubic bones in front.

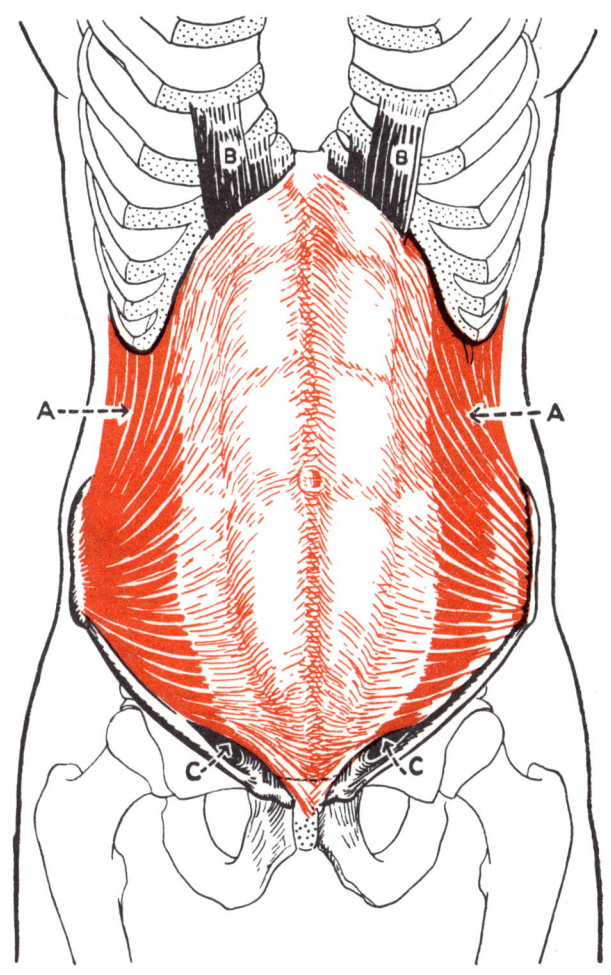

FIGURE 48—The internal oblique muscles of the abdomen
    A—Fibres of internal oblique
    B—Upper end of rectus abdominis
    C—Gap at the lower margin of internal oblique
       through which a rupture can occur

The middle layer of the abdomen is formed by the two *internal oblique* muscles (Figure 48), each lying under the corresponding external oblique muscle. Most of the fibres of the internal oblique run obliquely upward and inward, the line of pull of the muscle directly opposing that of the external oblique of the opposite side.

Origin: from the inguinal ligament, the crest of the ilium, and by a tendinous sheet from the lumbar vertebrae.

Insertion: by an aponeurosis into the aponeurosis of its fellow on the opposite side, into the crest of the pubis and the lower six ribs.

The arrangement of the aponeurosis of the internal oblique muscles is particularly interesting. The upper two thirds of each aponeurosis (Figure 49) splits into two layers as it approaches the front of the belly and reunites again shortly before the two aponeuroses join together at the midline. The two spaces thus left between the layers of the internal oblique are filled by the two recti abdominis muscles. This arrangement adds greatly to the strength of the anterior abdominal wall. The lower third of each aponeurosis does not split but passes in one layer in front of the rectus with the aponeurosis of the inner muscle layer (see Figure 50, B).

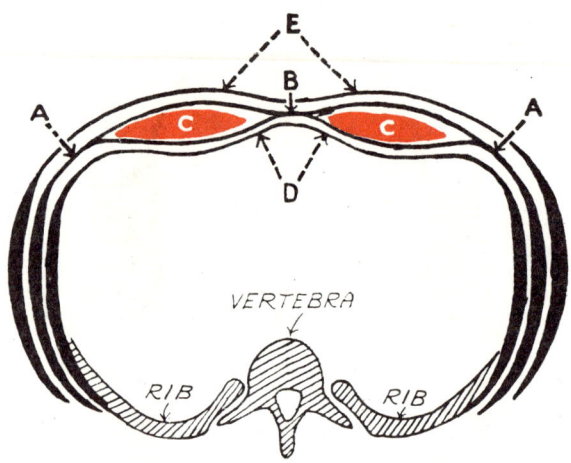

FIGURE 49—Section through the abdominal wall at level of navel (diagrammatic)
A—Aponeurosis of internal oblique
B—Midline
C—Rectus abdominis
D—Aponeuroses of transverse muscle
E—Aponeuroses of external oblique

The inner layer is formed by the two *transverse* muscles (Figures 50 and 51) which lie immediately beneath the internal oblique muscles. The fibres are directed horizontally and merge, like those of the oblique muscles into aponeuroses, each of which joins the combined tendinous insertion in the midline (Figure 49).

Origin: from the inguinal ligament, and the iliac crest, by tendinous bands from the lumbar vertebrae and from the lower six ribs.

Insertion: into the midline and the crest of the pubis.

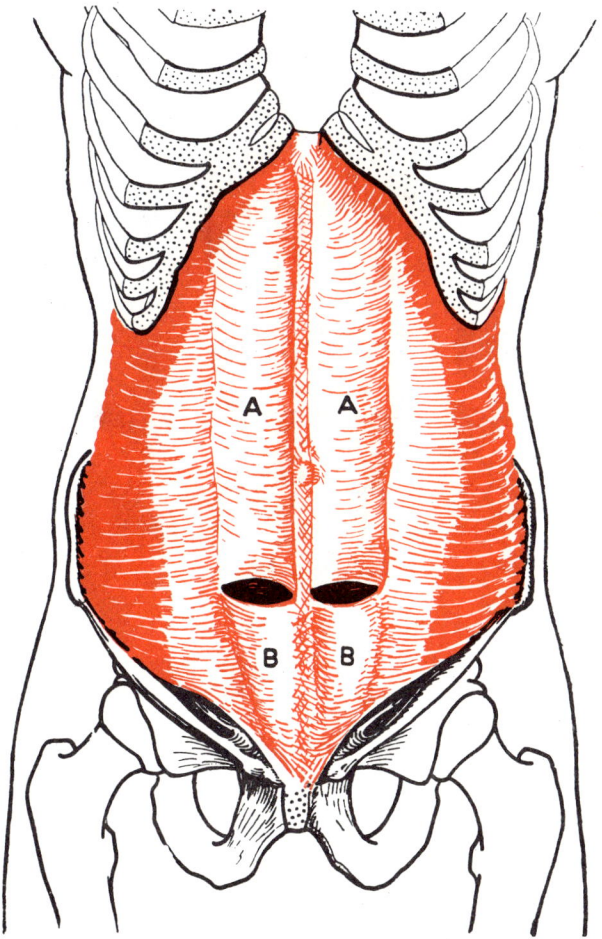

FIGURE 50—The transverse muscles of the abdomen showing the sheaths of the recti.
A—Aponeuroses forming posterior wall of rectus sheath
B—Aponeuroses forming anterior wall of rectus sheath

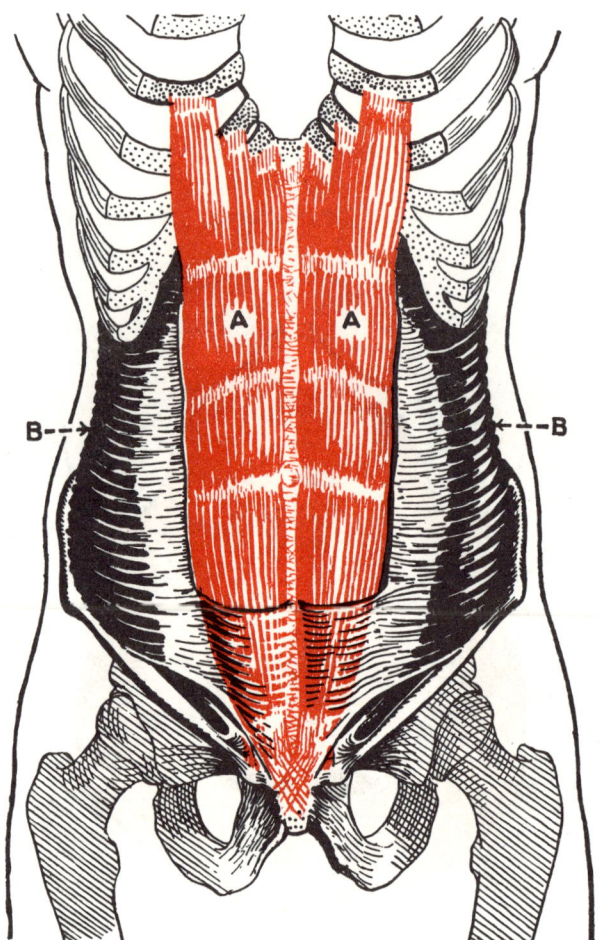

FIGURE 51
A—The rectus abdominis muscle
B—The transverse muscle

The *recti abdominis*. The anterior part of the abdominal wall is supported by the two recti abdominis (Figure 51) whose fibres run in a vertical direction.

Origin: from the crest of the pubis.

Insertion: into the cartilages of the fifth, sixth and seventh ribs.

Action of oblique, transverse and recti abdominis muscles: the fibres of the three flat muscles of the abdominal wall are arranged in a crisscross fashion (Figure 52); this arrangement not only provides strength without bulk, on the three ply principle, but allows a considerable variety of movements.

The two powerful pillars of the recti abdominis give additional strength in front where the pressure of the abdominal contents is most concentrated. The actions of these four pairs of muscles are of a somewhat complex nature. Their first and most important function is to act as a support for the abdominal contents and indirectly as accessory muscles of respiration. They are able to accommodate themselves to varying degrees of intra-abdominal pressure.

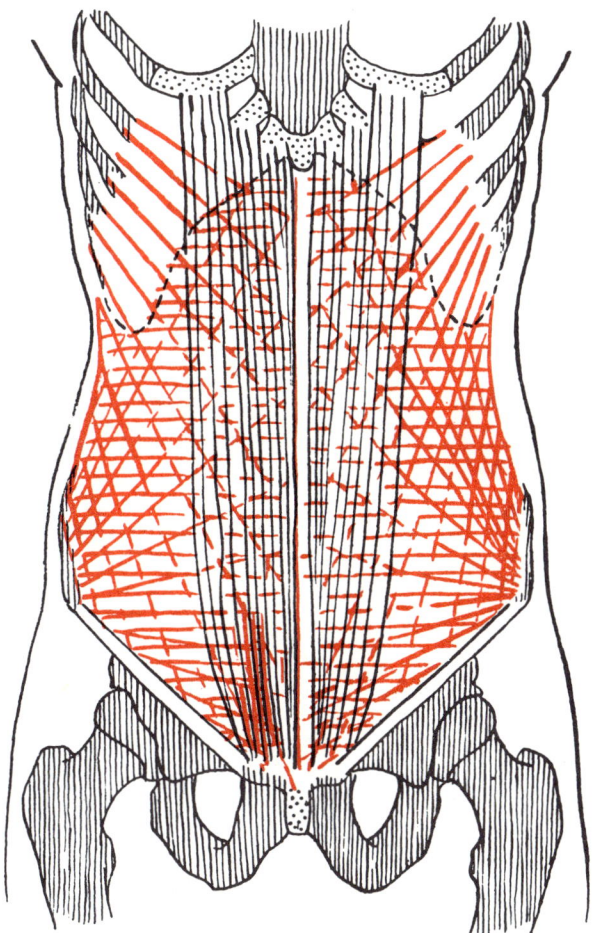

FIGURE 52—Diagram showing direction of fibres of the oblique, transverse and recti abdominis muscles

When, for example, a person who has been lying on his back, stands up, the increased pressure on the anterior abdominal wall is counteracted by these muscles; coughing, or straining as in defaecation, causes a considerable increase in pressure. The muscles, particularly in later life, may become unable to cope with these strains; they then stretch and weaken with the result that the abdominal contents become displaced downwards and forwards to form the well known corporation.

A similar state of affairs is brought about by paralysis of the abdominal muscles in certain cases of infantile paralysis. Such a patient, usually young, develops a pot belly with marked ballooning of the abdomen; he may be unable to maintain the fully erect position but stands with his pelvis tilted forward because the anterior abdominal muscles, particularly the recti, are unable to pull the front of the pelvis up into its normal position, against the pull of the muscles of the back.

The second function of the anterior and lateral abdominal muscles is to assist in maintaining erect and moving the vertebral column; the movements may be divided into:

(i) sideways bending of the vertebral column performed by the obliques and rectus of one side assisted by the posterior abdominal and spinal muscles of the same side;

(ii) rotation of the vertebral column; this movement is carried out by the external oblique of one side acting with the internal oblique of the opposite side, in conjunction with the rotator muscles of the spine;

(iii) flexion of the vertebral column performed mainly by the recti abdominis.

The actions of the muscles of the anterior abdominal wall are not in fact separated artificially as they must be for purposes of description; it is important to remember that all muscles, particularly those in groups, act in support of one another and seldom produce a single simple movement under natural conditions in life.

5. Muscles of the Posterior Abdominal Wall

The *quadratus lumborum* (the quadrilateral muscle of the lumbar region, Figure 53): each muscle lies at the side of and parallel to the lumbar portion of the vertebral column.

Origin: from the crest of the ilium.

Insertion: into the twelfth rib and transverse processes of the first four lumbar vertebrae.

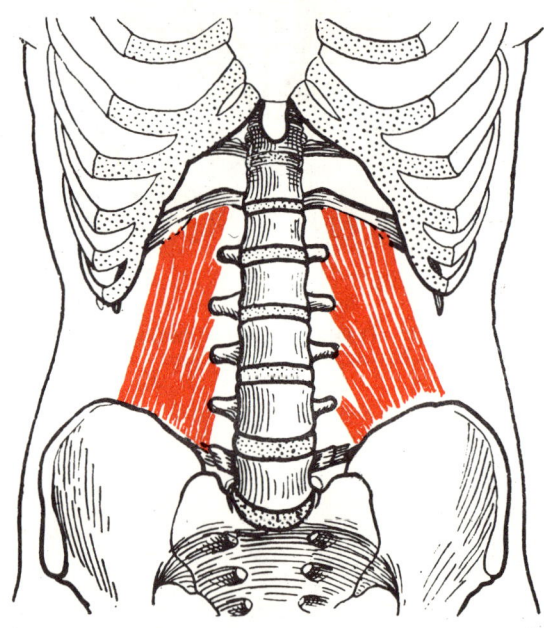

FIGURE 53—The quadrati lumborum

Action: the quadrati lumborum acting together draw down the last ribs and act as accessory muscles of respiration by helping to fix the origin of the diaphragm; each muscle acting alone bends the trunk to its own side. The remaining muscles of the posterior abdominal wall will be described with the muscles of the lower limb.

6. Muscles of the Pelvis (Figure 54)

There are four pairs of muscles forming the floor of the pelvis; only the *lavatores ani* will be described.

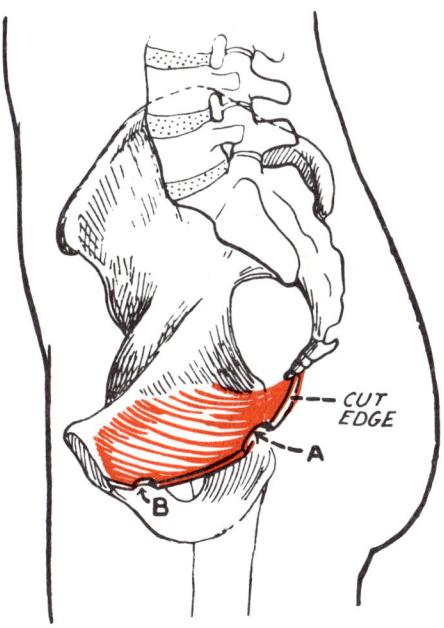

FIGURE 54—Section through pelvis viewed from the side showing the right levator ani (male)
A—Opening for anal canal
B—Opening for urethra

The *levator ani* (the elevating muscle of the anus) has a name which does not do full justice to its function; each is a broad thin muscle on either side of the floor of the pelvis; together they form what is called the *pelvic diaphragm*; the two muscles plug the gap in the pelvis and prevent the descent of the abdominal contents which would occur in their absence.

Origin: from the front, sides, and back of the pelvis.

Insertion: each muscle unites in the midline of the pelvic cavity with its fellow on the opposite side, leaving a gap for the *anal canal* and *urethra** in the male and for the vagina, urethra and the anal canal in the female.

Action: in addition to their important function of supporting the abdominal contents, they constrict the anal canal and raise the pelvic floor thus controlling defaecation.

*The urethra is the passage through which urine is expelled from the bladder.

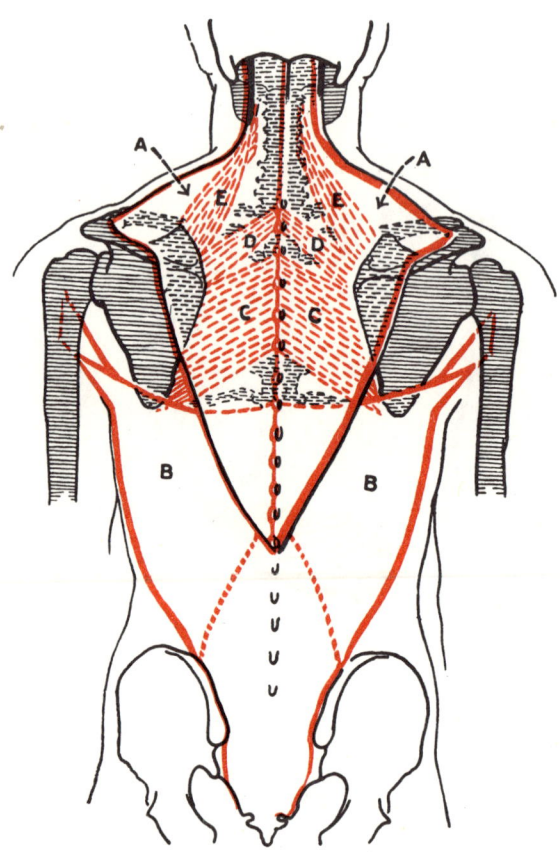

FIGURE 55—Muscles connecting the upper limbs to the vertebral column: viewed from behind (diagrammatic)

A—Trapezius
B—Latissimus dorsi
C—Rhomboideus major
D—Rhomboideus minor
E—Levator scapulae

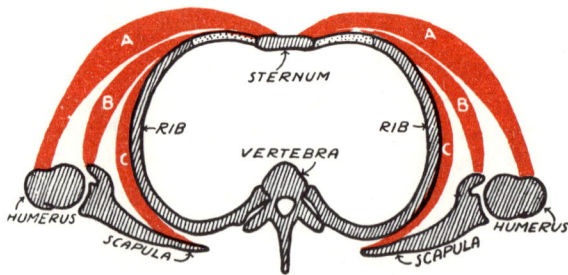

FIGURE 56—Section through the upper part of the thorax, viewed from above showing muscles connecting the thorax to the upper limbs (diagrammatic)

A—Pectoralis major
B—Pectoralis minor
C—Serratus anterior

MUSCLES OF THE UPPER LIMB
CLASSIFICATION

(1) Muscles Connecting the Vertebrae to the Upper Limb (Figure 55)

They lie on the posterior aspect of the thorax and are mainly concerned with movements of the shoulder girdle, with the exception of one muscle which moves the upper arm.

  (i) the *trapezius*;
  (ii) the *latissimus dorsi*;
  (iii) the *rhomboideus major and minor*;
  (iv) the *levator scapulae*.

(2) Muscles Connecting the Walls of the Thorax to the Upper Limb (Figure 56)

These three muscles are situated at the sides and front of the thorax; their main function is to draw the whole of the upper limb forward and inward and to rotate the scapula:

  (i) the *pectoralis major*;
  (ii) the *pectoralis minor*;
  (iii) the *serratus anterior*.

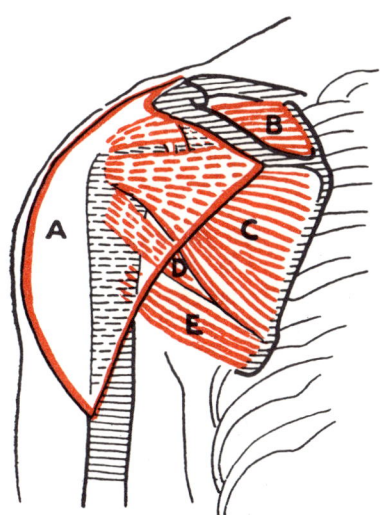

FIGURE 57—Muscles of the left shoulder girdle viewed from behind (diagrammatic)
A—Deltoid   C—Infraspinatus
B—Suprapinatus   D—Teres minor
E—Teres major.

(3) Muscles of the Shoulder Girdle (Figure 57)

These consist of one large muscle which covers the shoulder joint and five smaller muscles which pass from the scapula to the neck of the humerus. The function of these muscles is to move the arm and to control its movements at the shoulder joint:

  (i) the *deltoid*;
  (ii) the *supraspinatus*;
  (iii) the *infraspinatus* and *teres minor*;
  (iv) the *teres major*;
  (v) the *subscapularis*.

(4) Muscles of the Upper Arm

These may be classified as shown below.

The *anterior* group whose most important function is flexion of the elbow joint:
- (i) the *biceps brachialis*;
- (ii) the *brachialis*;
- (iii) the *coracobrachialis*.

The *posterior* muscle whose main function is extension of the elbow joint; this is the *triceps*.

(5) Muscles of the Forearm

It is necessary to know the actions rather than the names of the muscles of the forearm and they will therefore be classified according to function. They consist of:
- (i) flexors of the wrist, fingers and thumb;
- (ii) extensors of the wrist, fingers and thumb;
- (iii) rotators of the forearm.

(6) Muscles of the Hand

The muscles of the hand may be divided into two main groups;
- (i) the short, superficial muscles of the thumb and little finger;
- (ii) the deep muscles of the hand.

ARRANGEMENT AND ACTION

(1) Muscles Connecting the Vertebrae to the Upper Limb

(i) The *trapezius** (Figure 58): each muscle is broad, flat and triangular in shape: it lies immediately under the skin of the back. All its fibres converge toward the upper part of the shoulder.

Origin: from the back of the skull, the elastic ligament between the cervical spines, and the spinous processes of the seventh cervical and all the dorsal vertebrae.

Insertion: into the outer border of the clavicle, the acromion, and the spine of the scapula.

Action: the trapezius can elevate, depress or brace the shoulder backward. When the shoulders are fixed the trapezii, acting together, can draw the head backward; acting singly, the muscle can bend the head sideways; it has a very important part to play in controlling the elevation of the arm above shoulder level.

*It is called trapezius because the two muscles together roughly form a trapezium, a four-sided figure with no two sides parallel.

(ii) The *latissimus dorsi* (the broadest muscle of the back, Figure 58): this is a large triangular muscle which covers the lumbar and lower half of the thoracic region; its fibres are directed upward and outward and converge toward the armpit.

Origin: from the crest of the ilium, the sacrum, the spinous processes of the lumbar and lower six dorsal vertebrae, the lower four ribs and sometimes from the inferior angle of the scapula.

Insertion: by a single tendon into the inner and anterior surface of the humerus about two inches below the head; as may be seen in Figure 58, the muscle twists on itself at C so that the upper fibres are inserted below the lower fibres.

Action: its main action is to bring the arm from an abducted position to the side of the body; in its reverse action, it pulls the body up to the arm; it is also an extensor of the upper arm.

The latissimus dorsi assists, by its attachment to the lower four ribs, in fixing the origin of the diaphragm when the latter is called upon to contract more powerfully than usual, as, for example, during coughing, sneezing, and straining in defaecation.

The upper part of this muscle passes across the lower third of the scapula and helps to maintain the close proximity of this bone to the chest wall, when pushing movements are performed.

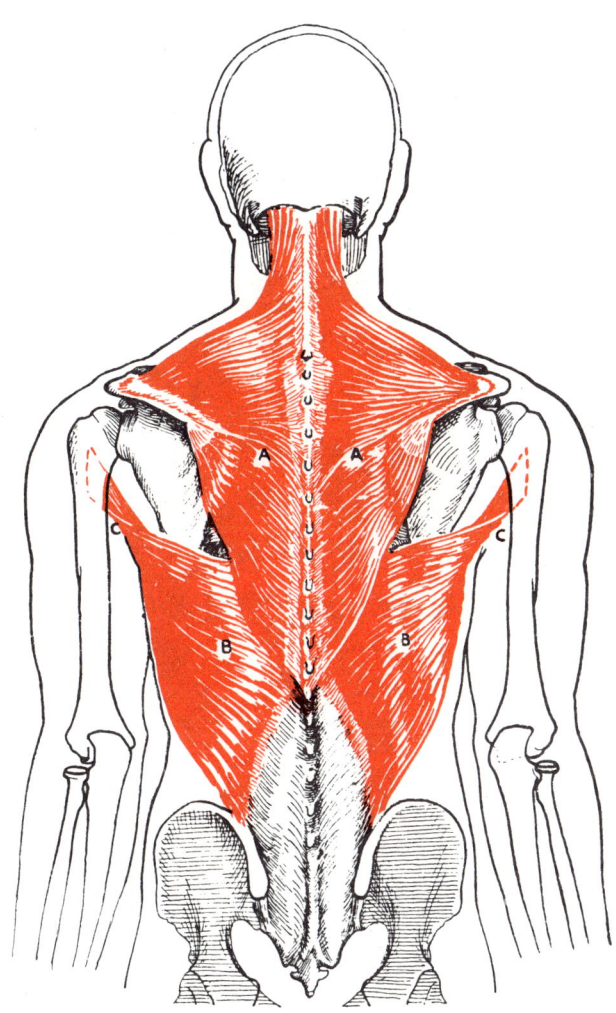

FIGURE 58

A—Trapezius
B—Latissimus dorsi
C—Twisting of muscle fibres near insertion

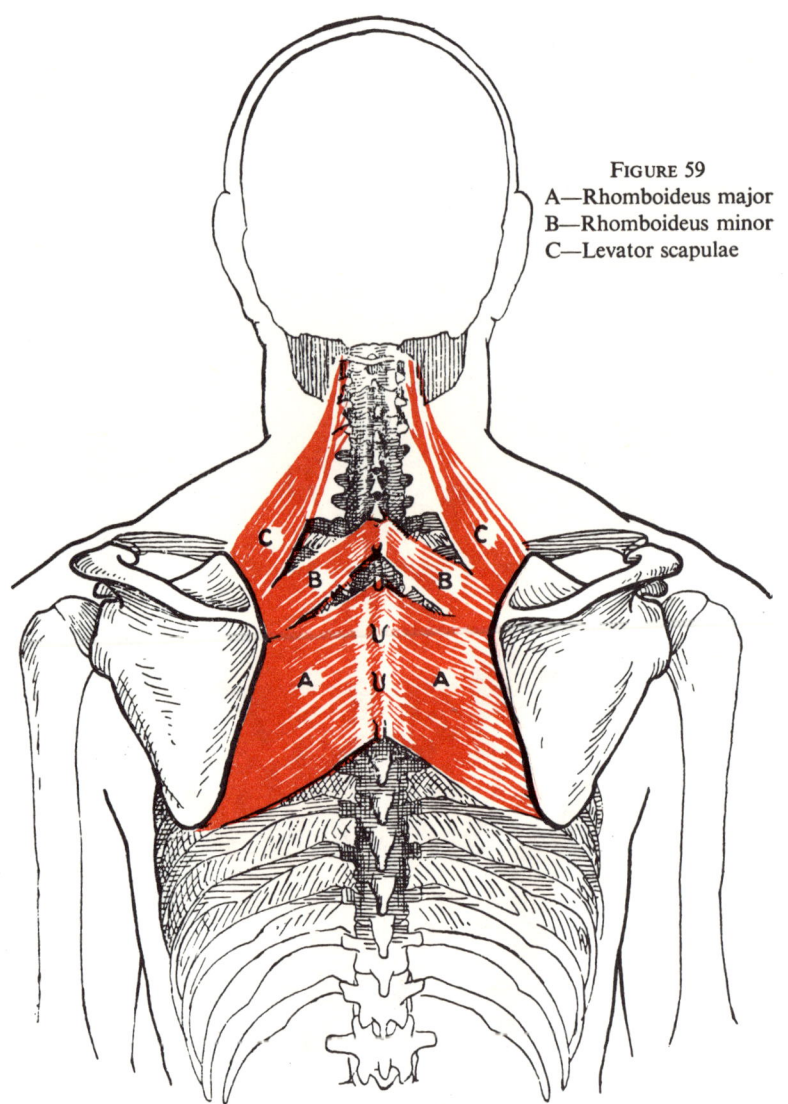

FIGURE 59
A—Rhomboideus major
B—Rhomboideus minor
C—Levator scapulae

(iii) The *rhomboideus major and minor* (the large and small rhomboid shaped muscles, Figure 59): these two muscles lie between the scapula and the upper part of the vertebral column.

Origins: the major, from the spinous processes of the second to the fifth dorsal vertebrae, and the minor, from the spinous processes of the seventh cervical and first dorsal vertebrae.

Insertions: into the inner or vertebral border of the scapula.

Actions: the two muscles have a similar action in drawing the lower angle of the scapula upward and inward, thus depressing the point of the shoulder.

(iv) The *levator scapulae* (the elevating muscle of the scapula, Figure 59): this muscle lies underneath the trapezius; its fibres are directed upward and inward towards the base of the skull.

Origin: from the transverse processes of the first four cervical vertebrae.
Insertion: into the upper and inner border of the scapula.
Action: this muscle helps to elevate the scapula when the cervical part

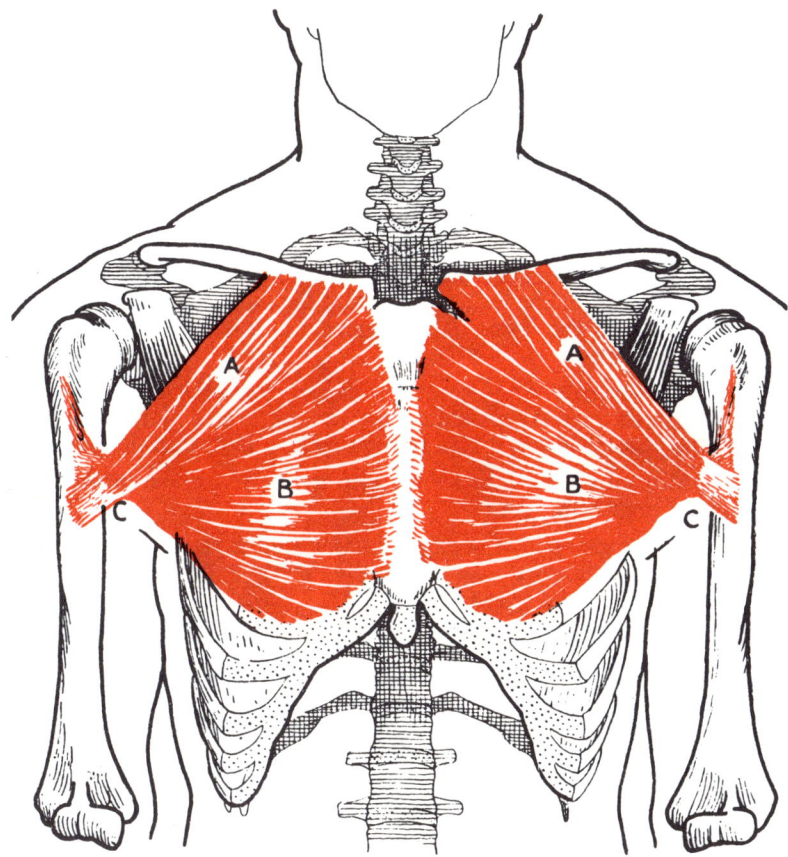

FIGURE 60
A—Clavicular part of pectoralis major
B—Sternal part of pectoralis major
C—Twisting of muscle fibres near the insertion of sternal part

of the vertebral column remains fixed; when the shoulder is fixed, each muscle bends the head and neck to its own side.

(2) Muscles connecting the Walls of the Thorax to the Upper Limb

(i) The *pectoralis major* (the large muscle of the chest, Figure 60): this is a broad, thick triangular muscle which stretches across the front of the chest from the sternum to the armpit.

Origin: the upper portion of this muscle arises from the inner third of the clavicle, and the lower portion from the sternum and the cartilages of the upper six ribs.

Insertion: the fibres all converge to be inserted into the humerus immediately in front of the insertion of the latissimus dorsi; those fibres arising from the sternum and costal cartilages twist upon themselves at C before they reach their insertion, so that the upper fibres of the sternal portion of this muscle are inserted below the lower fibres.

Action: the chief action is adduction but the muscle also produces internal rotation and flexion of the upper arm.

The upper or clavicular portion of the muscle completes the movement of adduction initiated by the lower or sternal portion. The reason for this is that the maximum pull on a lever is obtained when the line of pull is directly at right angles to the arm of the lever. In Figure 61, the line AB in the left-hand diagram representing the pull of the sternal portion of the pectoralis major, is at right angles to the humerus and therefore exerts a greater pull than the clavicular portion.

When the arm is adducted further towards the opposite shoulder as in the right-hand diagram, the line DC, representing the pull of the clavicular portion, is at right angles to the humerus and therefore able to exert a greater pull than the sternal portion.

Briefly, all movements of adduction or internal rotation, outside an imaginary vertical line EF, through the shoulder joint, are performed mainly by the sternal portion of the pectoralis major, and inside this line, by the clavicular portion.

Flexion or forward elevation of the upper arm is performed by the clavicular portion of the pectoralis major.

The latissimus dorsi and the pectoralis major are the most important climbing muscles of the upper limb.

(ii) The *pectoralis minor* (the small muscle of the chest, Figure 62): this small triangular muscle lies underneath the outer part of the pectoralis major.

Origin: from the outer surfaces of the third, fourth and fifth ribs.

Insertion: into the coracoid process of the scapula.

Action: it assists in drawing the scapula forward round the chest wall; it also depresses the point of the shoulder.

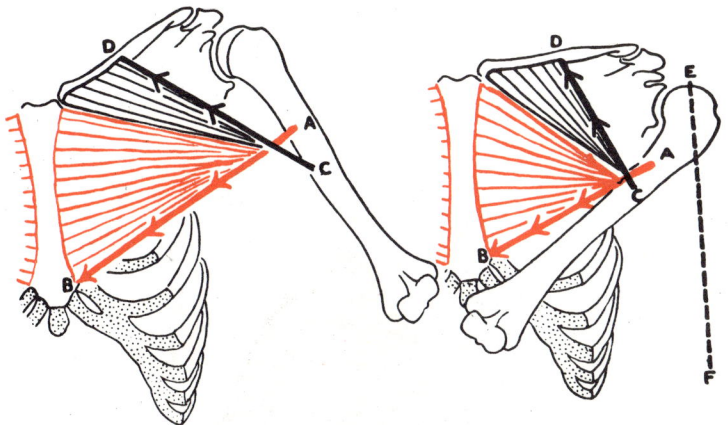

FIGURE 61

Diagram showing position of maximum pull of sternal portion of left pectoralis major

Diagram showing position of maximum pull of clavicular portion of left pectoralis major

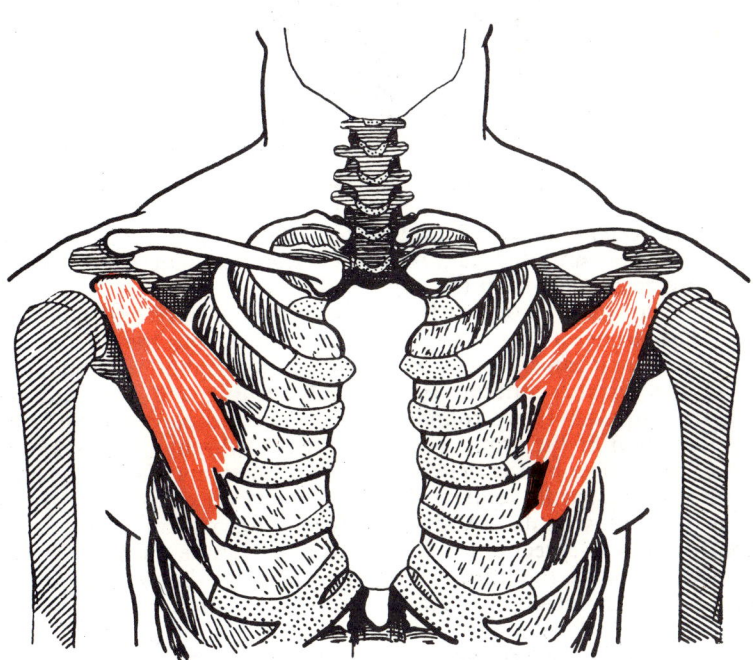

FIGURE 62—The pectoralis minor

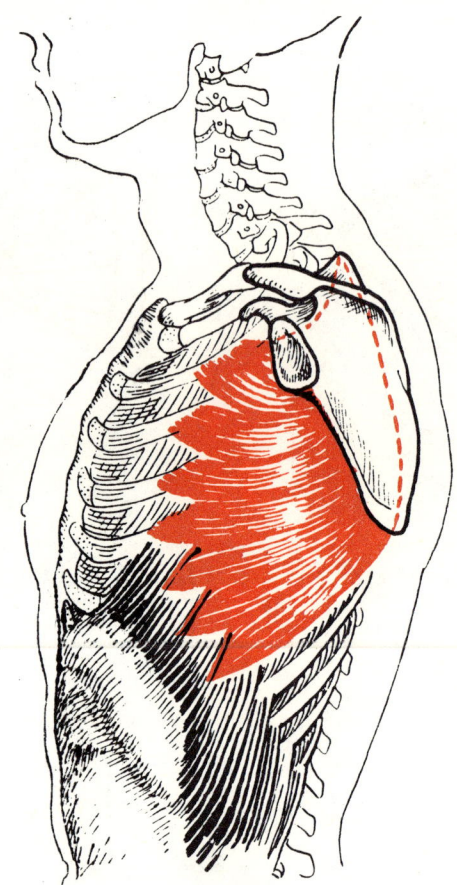

FIGURE 63—The left serratus anterior

(iii) The *serratus anterior** (Figure 63): this muscle covers most of the side of the chest wall and its posterior portion lies underneath the scapula.

Origin: by fleshy slips from the upper eight ribs.

Insertion: along the under surface of the inner or vertebral border of the scapula. The strongest part of the muscle is inserted into the inferior angle of the scapula where it can exert its greatest pull at the point of maximum leverage.

Action: the serratus anterior is the chief pushing and punching muscle; it draws the scapula forward round the chest wall and plays a most important part in abduction of the arm. The arm is moved through the first 90 or 100 degrees of abduction by the deltoid and the smaller muscles of the shoulder, while the shoulder girdle remains fixed by the action of the serratus and the trapezius on the scapula. Abduction from approximately the horizontal position to one 45 degrees above it, is performed by the serratus anterior and trapezius which rotate the scapula while the shoulder joint remains fixed by the deltoid. When this position is reached, further rotation of the scapula does not occur and the deltoid cannot pull the arm up to the vertical position because the highest point of the humerus is impinging upon the acromion (Figure 91). The humerus must therefore be externally rotated and the limb can then be brought into the vertical position by further movement at the shoulder joint by the action mainly of the anterior fibres of the deltoid.

*This muscle is so called because its origin from the ribs is serrated or notched like the teeth of a saw. (There is also a small muscle, the serratus posterior, which will not be described)

If the serratus anterior is paralysed, the inner border and especially the inferior angle of the scapula, tilt away from the ribs and protrude backward; any attempt to push against a wall makes this deformity even more prominent, and gives a peculiar winged appearance to the back. Naturally, abduction of the arm above the horizontal position is not possible in these circumstances.

3. Muscles of the Shoulder

(i) The *deltoid** (Figure 64): this thick triangular muscle covers the shoulder joint in the manner shown in Figure 64. From the point of view of function, its fibres may be divided roughly into anterior, middle, and posterior fibres.

Origin: from the outer third of the clavicle, the acromion, and the spine of the scapula.

Insertion: the fibres converge into a single tendon which is inserted into the outer surface of the humerus about halfway down its shaft.

Action: the chief action is abduction of the arm from the side to approximately the horizontal position; it acts most strongly between the range of 15 to 90 degrees of abduction; this action is performed mainly by its middle fibres. The anterior fibres draw the upper arm forward (flexion) and bring it into the vertical position above the head; the posterior fibres draw the upper arm backward (extension).

*It is called deltoid because it has the triangular shape of the Greek capital 'Δ' or *delta*, represented by an equilateral triangle.

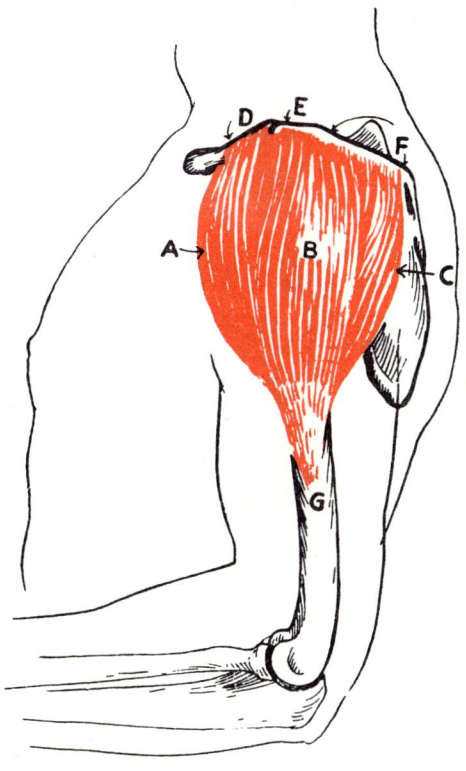

FIGURE 64—The left deltoid: side view
A—Anterior fibres   D—Clavicle
B—Middle fibres   E—Acromion
C—Posterior fibres   F—Spine of scapula
G—Insertion of deltoid

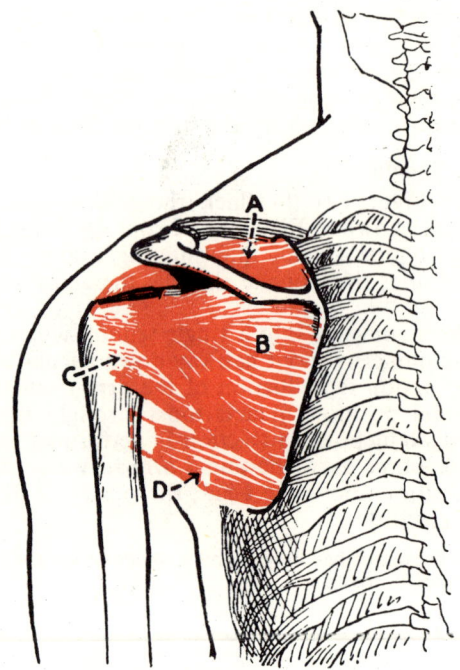

FIGURE 65—The left supraspinatus, infraspinatus, teres major and minor
A—Supraspinatus
B—Infraspinatus
C—Teres minor
D—Teres major

FRONT VIEW

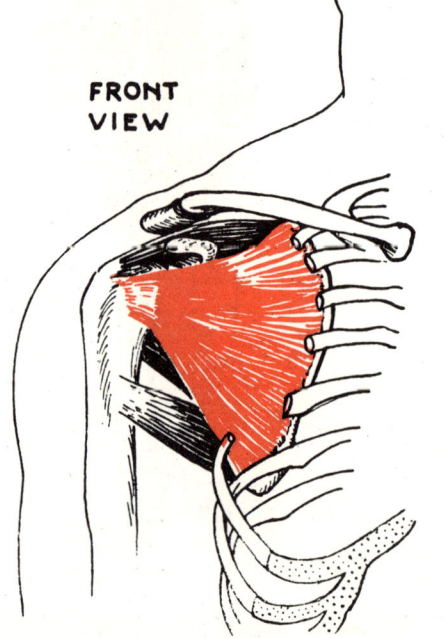

FIGURE 66—The right subscapularis muscle. It covers the whole undersurface of the scapula. (Portions af the ribs have been cut away)

(ii) The *supraspinatus* (the muscle above the spine of the scapula, Figure 65): this muscle lies in the groove above the spine of the scapula and its tendon crosses the top of the shoulder joint.

Origin: from the upper part of the body of the scapula.

Insertion: into the highest point on the neck of the humerus.*

Action: it plays the chief part in moving the arm through the first 10 or 15 degrees of abduction.

(iii) The *infraspinatus* (the muscle below the spine of the scapula, Figure 65) and the *teres minor* (the small rounded muscle, Figure 65): these two muscles are situated below the spine of the scapula and their tendons pass behind the shoulder joint.

Origins: from the body of the scapula.

Insertions: into the neck of the humerus, the insertion of the infraspinatus being immediately above that of the teres minor and below that of the supraspinatus.

Actions: both muscles rotate the upper arm externally and assist in adduction (drawing the arm to the side).

(iv) The *teres major* (the large rounded muscle, Figure 65): this thick, somewhat rounded muscle, crosses from the inferior angle of the scapula, behind the armpit, to the upper part of the humerus in front.

Origin: from the inferior angle of the scapula.

Insertion: into the inner and anterior surface of the humerus about one inch below the head.

Action: the muscle rotates the upper arm internally and draws it inward and backward.

(v) The *subscapularis* (the muscle lying under the scapula, Figure 66): this muscle is situated on the under surface of the body of the scapula, between that bone and the ribs.

Origin: from the flat under surface of the scapula.

Insertion: into the front of the neck of the humerus.

Action: it is chiefly an internal rotator of the arm, but when the arm is raised it helps to adduct the arm to the side.

The tendons of all the smaller muscles of the shoulder joint are closely blended with the joint capsule and thus form a very strong tendinous cuff which envelops the top and sides of the head of the humerus.

During abduction of the shoulder, these muscles contract and hold the head of the humerus firmly in apposition to the glenoid fossa and thus counteract the natural tendency of the head of the humerus to ride upward over the joint margin; as soon as the head of the humerus is held down firmly, the movement of abduction by the supraspinatus can be started.

*This point is called the *greater tuberosity*.

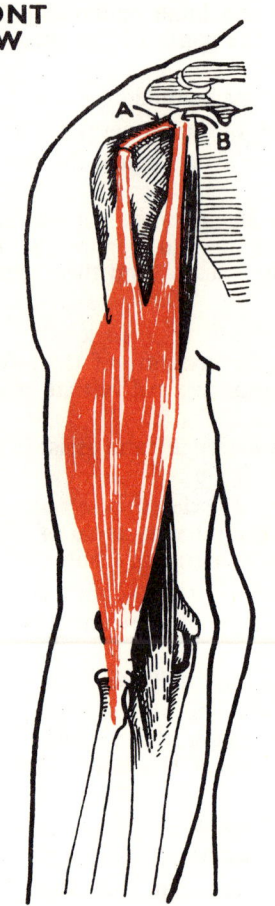
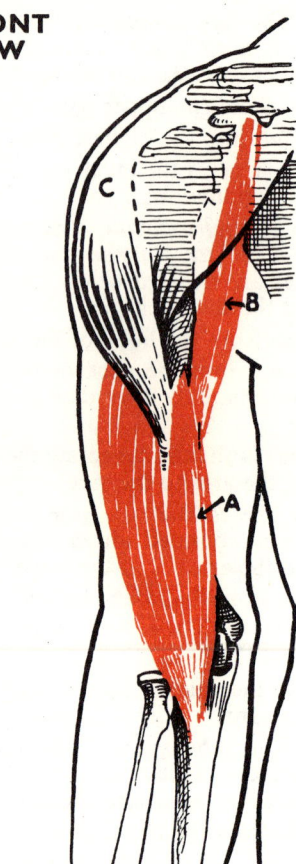

FIGURE 67—The right biceps brachialis
A—Long head (marked by arrow)
B—Short head (marked by arrow)

FIGURE 68 A—Brachialis
B—Coracobrachialis
C—Deltoid

4. Muscles of the Upper Arm
Anterior group

(i) The *biceps brachialis* (the two-headed muscle of the arm, Figure 67): this muscle lies along the front of the forearm.

Origin: by two tendons or heads; one called the *long* head arises from a point just above the glenoid fossa, the other, the *short* head from the coracoid process of the scapula.

Insertion: into the inner aspect of the radius about three quarters of an inch below its head.

Action: it is primarily a supinator of the forearm and secondarily a flexor of the elbow joint.

The tendon of the long head of the biceps acts as an accessory ligament of the shoulder joint and is closely blended into the joint capsule.

(ii) The *brachialis* (the muscle of the arm, Figure 68): this muscle lies over the lower end of the humerus and the front of the elbow joint.

Origin: from the front of the lower half of the humerus.

Insertion: into the upper end of the ulna about half an inch below the elbow joint.

Action: it is the chief flexor muscle of the elbow joint.

(iii) The *coracobrachialis* (the arm muscle attached to the coracoid process, Figure 68): this is a small, straight muscle situated on the inner side of the upper arm.
Origin: from the coracoid process.
Insertion: into the inner side of the humerus about midway down its shaft.
Action: this muscle is a weak adductor and flexor of the upper arm.

Posterior muscle

The *triceps* (the three-headed muscle, Figure 69): this muscle covers the whole of the back of the humerus.

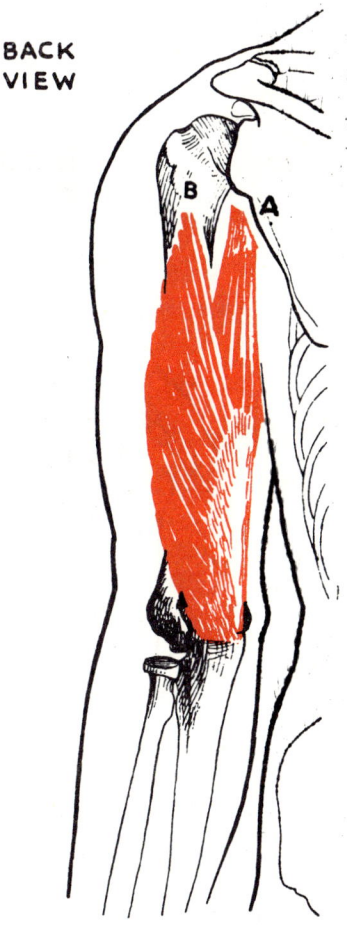

FIGURE 69—Triceps
A—Long head
B—Lateral head covering the medial head

Origin: by three separate origins or *heads*: the *long* head arises from immediately below the glenoid fossa, and the other two heads, a *lateral* and a *medial*, from the middle of the posterior aspect of the humerus. They blend into one tendon.
Insertion: into the olecranon process.
Action: extension of the elbow; it also assists in adduction of the upper arm.

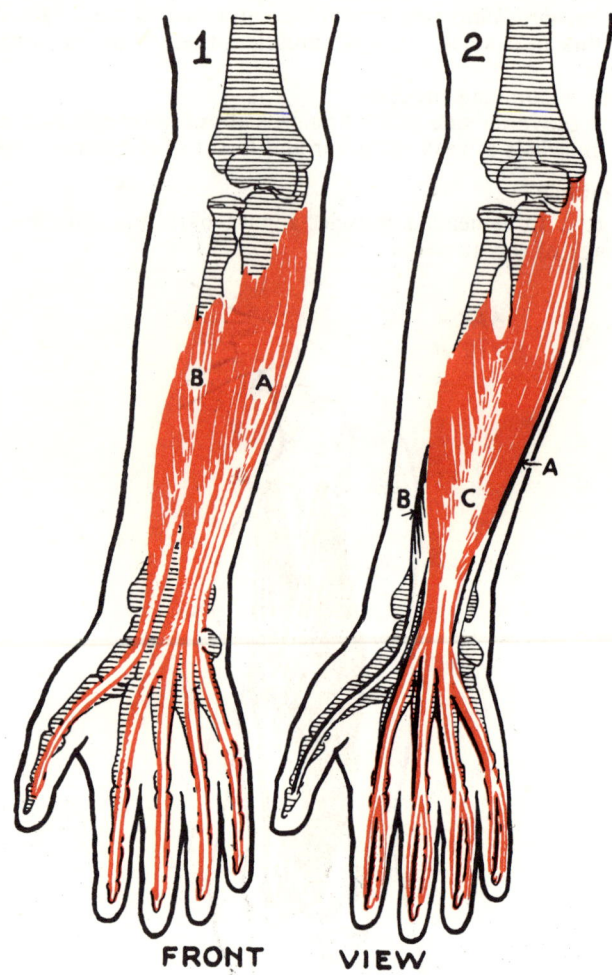

FIGURE 70—The long flexors of the fingers and thumb
(Right forearm)
1 Deep group of flexors
2—Superficial group of flexors
A—Deep flexor of fingers   C—Superficial flexor of the
B—Flexor of the thumb   fingers

5. Muscles of the Forearm

(i) *The Flexor Group* (Figure 70).

The long flexors of the fingers and thumb: these muscles lie mainly on the ulnar side of the front of the forearm. They are more powerful than the opposing extensor muscles because they are the chief muscles of gripping; the extensors are seldom called upon to do work against active resistance, their chief function being to open the fist and extend the fingers.

The long muscles of the fingers perform the strong, coarser movements of the fingers whereas the short muscles in the hand, which will be mentioned later, perform the movements of precision.

Origins: from the bony prominence or condyle on the inner side of the lower end of the humerus, and from the fronts of the shafts of the radius and ulna.

Insertions: into the last two phalanges of the fingers and thumb.

Actions: flexion of the fingers and thumb; they assist in flexion of the wrist.

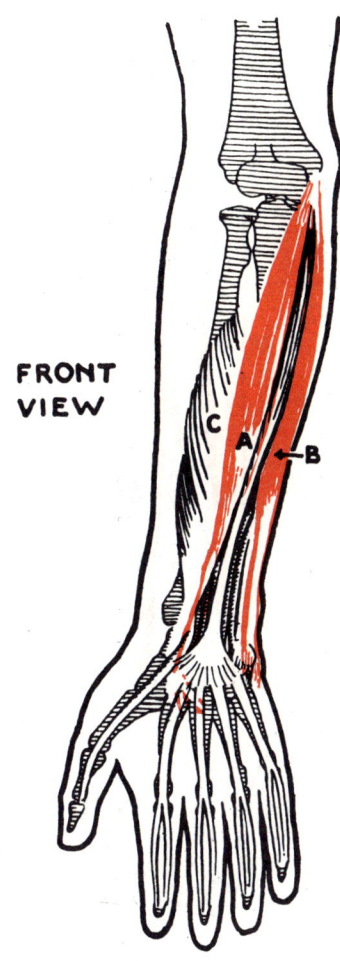

FIGURE 71

A
B } Flexors of the wrist
C—Part of superficial flexor of the fingers

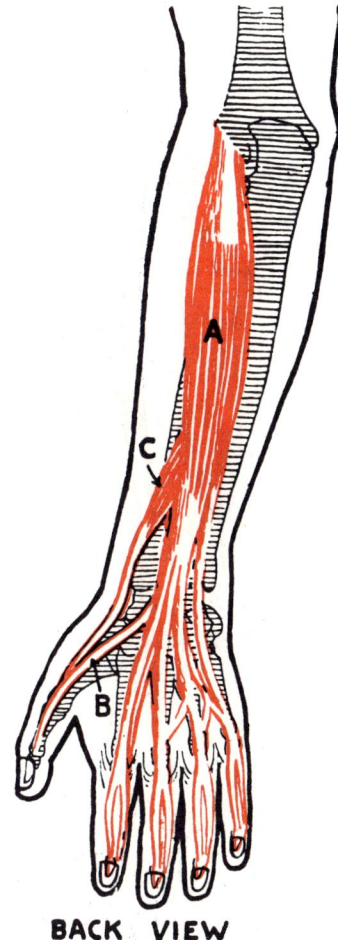

FIGURE 72

A—Long extensor of the fingers
B—Long extensor of the thumb
C—Long abductor of the thumb

Flexors of the wrist (Figure 71): there are two muscles whose main function is flexion of the wrist. They arise from the inner condyle of the lower end of the humerus and from the ulna and are inserted into the carpus and the bases of the metacarpals.

Actions: flexion of the wrist when acting together. When acting separately, the muscle B^2 in Figure 74, inserted on the ulnar side of the carpus performs the movement of ulnar deviation (see page 29) and the other, B^1, on the radial side, radial deviation.

(ii) *The Extensor Group* (Figure 72).

The long extensors of the fingers and thumb: the extensor group is situated on the radial side and the back of the forearm.

Origins: from the bony prominence or condyle on the outer side of the lower end of the humerus, and from the posterior aspects of the shafts of the radius and ulna.

Insertions: into the last two phalanges of the fingers and thumb.

Actions: extension of the fingers and thumb; they assist in extension of the wrist.

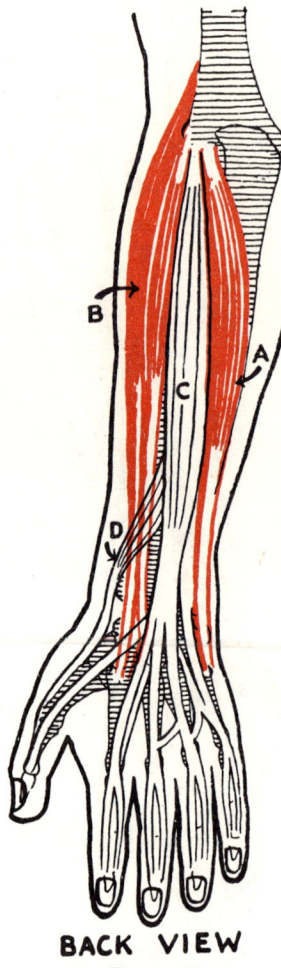
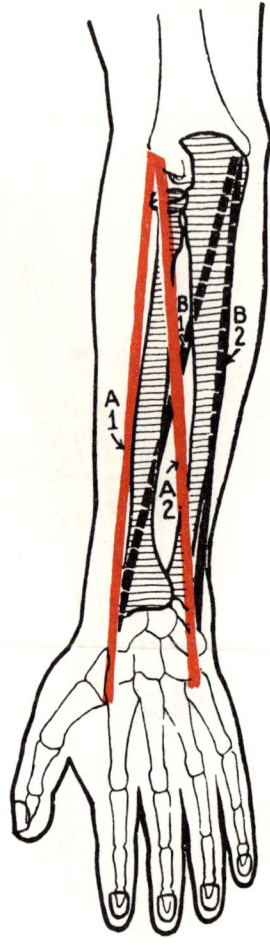

BACK VIEW

FIGURE 73
A and B—Extensors of the wrist
C—Long extensor of the fingers
D—Long abductor of the thumb

FIGURE 74—Diagrammatic representation of the flexors and extensors of the wrist
A^1, A^2—Extensors
B^1, B^2—Flexors

Extensors of the wrist (Figure 73): there are three; they arise mainly from the outer condyle of the lower end of the humerus and are inserted into the bases of the metacarpals on the back of the hand, one on the ulnar and the others on the radial border.

Actions: acting together they dorsiflex or extend the wrist; acting separately the muscle B in Figure 73 produces radial deviation, and the muscle A, ulnar deviation.

In these movements each is assisted by the corresponding flexor of the wrist. In Figure 74 the extensor A^1 works with the flexor B^1 to produce radial deviation, and A^2 with B^2 to produce ulnar deviation.

An injury to the nerve which supplies the extensor group of muscles causes a condition known as *wrist drop*. A patient suffering from it is unable to extend the wrist or fingers and cannot move his thumb dorsally from the palm of his hand. The condition is relatively common because the nerve supply of the extensor groups is particularly exposed to injury in cases of fracture of the humerus. It also occurs in cases of lead poisoning and as a result of prolonged and excessive indulgence in alcohol.

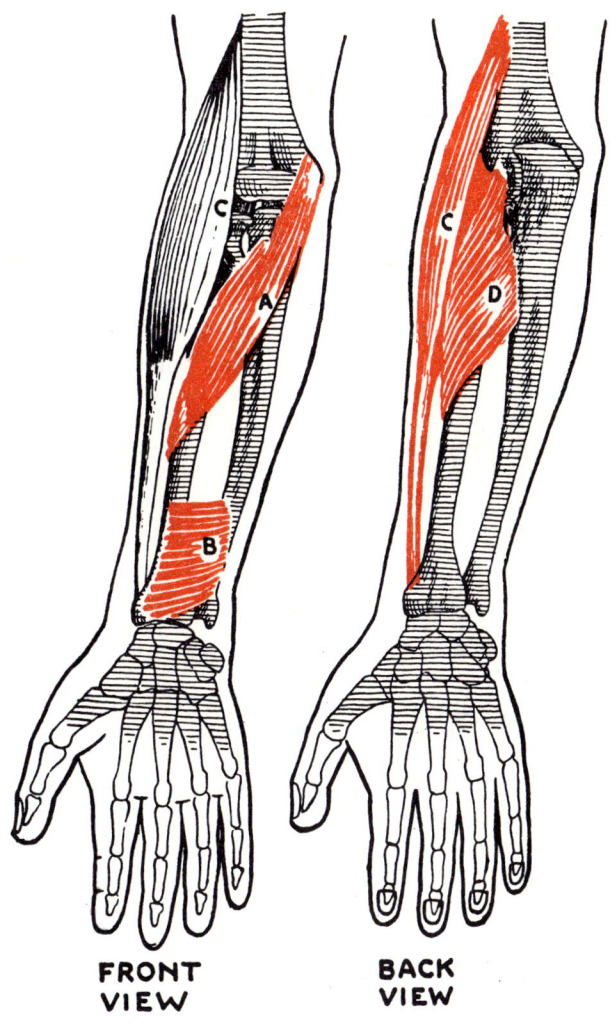

FIGURE 75—Rotators of the forearm
A—Pronator teres   C—Brachioradialis
B—Pronator quadratus   D—Short supinator

(iii) *The Rotators of the Forearm.*
    (a) The *pronator teres* and *pronator quadratus*;
    (b) The *brachioradialis* and *short supinator*.

The *pronator teres* (the rounded muscle of pronation. Figure 75): this muscle lies among the flexor group.

Origin: from the common flexor origin on the lower end of the humerus and from the upper end of the ulna.

Insertion: into the outer aspect of the middle of the shaft of the radius.

Action: its chief action is pronation, which it performs by rolling the lower part of the radius round the ulna. Its subsidiary action is flexion of the elbow joint.

    The *pronator quadratus* (the rectangular muscle of pronation. Figure 75): this muscle arises from the lower end of the ulna and is inserted into the lower end of the radius; it acts as a pronator only.

The *brachioradialis* (Figure 75) is a flexor of the elbow though it is situated in the extensor group.

Origin: from the outer part of the lower end of the humerus.

Insertion: into the outer aspect of the lower end of the radius.

Action: it is a flexor of the elbow and acts most strongly when the forearm is in the position midway between full supination and full pronation.

The *short supinator* (Figure 75) is a small but important muscle situated between the upper ends of the radius and ulna.

Origin: from the outer side of the elbow joint and the outer aspect of the upper end of the ulna.

Insertion: into the outer surface of the upper third of the radius.

Action: it assists the biceps in performing supination of the forearm. Supination is an extremely important component of complex movement of the wrist; it is essential in using a screwdriver. Loss of the power of pronation, however, can be overcome to a certain extent by abducting the arm at the shoulder which brings the forearm and hand into a position of greater pronation; there are no such movements by which limitation of supination can be overcome.

6. The Small Muscles of the Hand (Figure 76).

These are (i) the *superficial* muscles at the base of the thumb and little finger, and (ii) the *deep* muscles between the metacarpal bones and between the tendons of the hand.

The muscles of the thumb are among the most important in the whole of the upper limb; they bring the thumb into apposition with any one of the four fingers and thus make precise grasping movements possible. A hand without a thumb or with paralysis of the thumb muscles may be compared with a pair of pliers which has lost one of its jaws. The loss of one or even two fingers, however, does not impair the usefulness of the hand nearly as much as might be expected. The muscles of the little finger are relatively unimportant.

Both groups of muscles arise from the bones and ligaments of the carpus and are inserted into the phalanges of the thumb and little finger. The thumb muscles have four separate actions:

(1) they draw the thumb across the palm of the hand to oppose the other fingers; this movement is *opposition*;

(2) they move it directly away from the palm of the hand in a plane at right angles to its surface; this movement is *abduction*;

(3) they press the adjacent margins of the thumb and index finger together; this movement is called *adduction;*

(4) they flex the joints of the thumb.

The deep muscles of the hand are the four *lumbrical* muscles, so named on account of their likeness to earthworms, and the seven *interosseous* muscles which lie between the metacarpals.

The action of the interossei is to straighten the phalangeal joints, bend the metacarpo-phalangeal joints and to spread the fingers and to draw them together.

The condition called *claw hand* may occur if the nerve which supplies these deep muscles is injured; in this condition the joints become fixed in positions shown in Figure 78. Comparison of Figures 77 and 78 shows that the joints flexed in Figure 77 are extended in Figure 78 and vice versa.

The reason for this is that the muscles which extend the joints between the metacarpals and the phalanges and which flex the interphalangeal joints are now completely unopposed and remain in a state of chronic contraction.

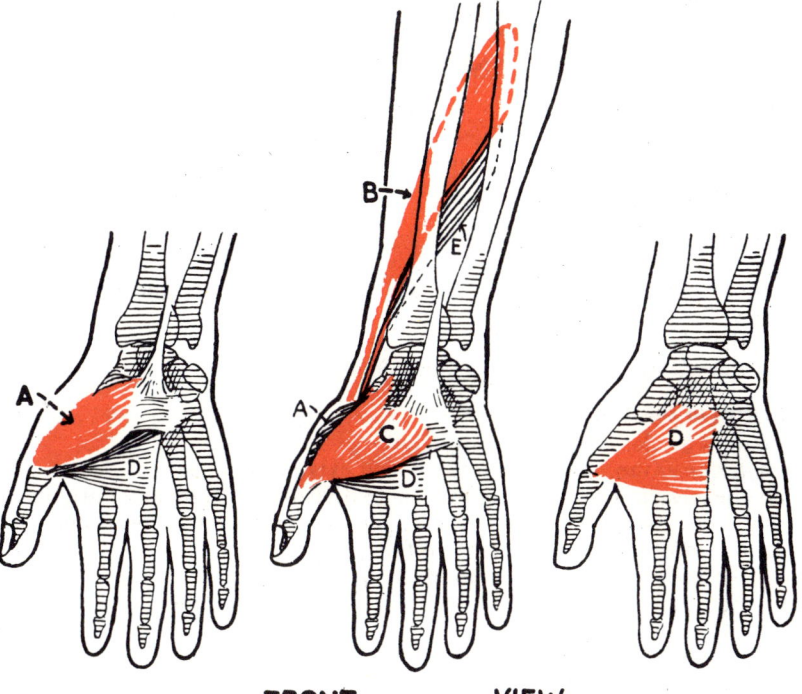

FRONT VIEW

FIGURE 76—The superficial muscles of the thumb
(The long abductor and short extensor of the thumb are shown in this group because they belong to it functionally)
A—Muscle of opposition
B—Long abductor (short abductor not shown)
C—Short flexor
D—Adductor
E—Short extensor

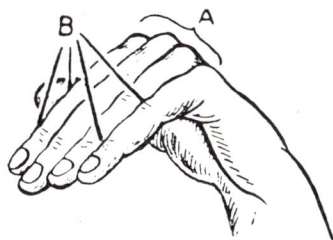

FIGURE 77—Position of the hand when the interossei and lumbricals are contracting
A—Joints flexed by the lumbricals
B—Joints extended by the interossei

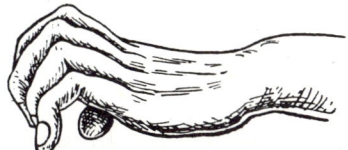

FIGURE 78—Claw hand
Position of the hand when the interossei and lumbricals are paralysed

MUSCLES OF THE LOWER LIMB
CLASSIFICATION

1. Muscles of the Pelvis

There are two muscles which lie on the posterior wall of the abdomen which act upon the lower limb. Their main action is flexion of the thigh:
    (i) the *psoas*;
    (ii) the *iliacus*.

2. Muscles of the Buttocks

The three muscles of the buttocks are mainly extensors and abductors of the thigh:
    (i) the *gluteus maximus*;
    (ii) the *gluteus medius* and *gluteus minimus*.

3. Muscles of the Thigh

These may be classified as shown below.
The *anterior* group, mainly muscles which extend the knee:
    (i) the *quadriceps*, which has four large divisions with separate origins and a combined insertion. The action is mainly extension of the knee. It is by far the most important muscle in this group;
    (ii) the *sartorius*, which lies upon the quadriceps;
    (iii) the *tensor fasciae latae* which is of some importance as a muscle of posture.
The last two muscles are not extensors of the knee, but are included in this group for convenience of description.
The *posterior* group, muscles which flex the knee and extend the hip;
    (i) the *biceps femoris*;
    (ii) the *semimembranosus* and *semitendinosus*.
The *internal* group of three muscles which adduct the thigh on the pelvis:
    the *adductores longus, magnus* and *brevis*.

4. Muscles of the Leg

The muscles of the leg may also be divided into three main groups.
The *anterior* group, which is concerned mainly with the extension of the five toes and dorsiflexion of the foot.
    (i) the *long extensors of the toes*;
    (ii) the *anterior tibial muscle*.
The *posterior* group containing flexors of the toes and plantar flexors of the ankle:
    (i) the *long flexors of the toes*;
    (ii) the *posterior tibial* muscle;
    (iii) the *gastrocnemius* and the *soleus*.
The *external* group containing muscles whose main function is eversion:
    the *peroneus longus* and *peroneus brevis*.

5. Muscles of the Foot

There are four layers of small muscles in the foot and though their function is extremely important, their general anatomical arrangement will not be set out in detail.

ARRANGEMENT AND ACTION

1. Muscles of the Pelvis

    (i) The *psoas** *major* (Figure 79) is a long muscle which is situated at the back of the abdomen; its lower portion crosses the inner surface of the upper part of the innominate bone and passes out over the rim of the pelvis into the upper part of the thigh.

*Psoas means "of the loin."

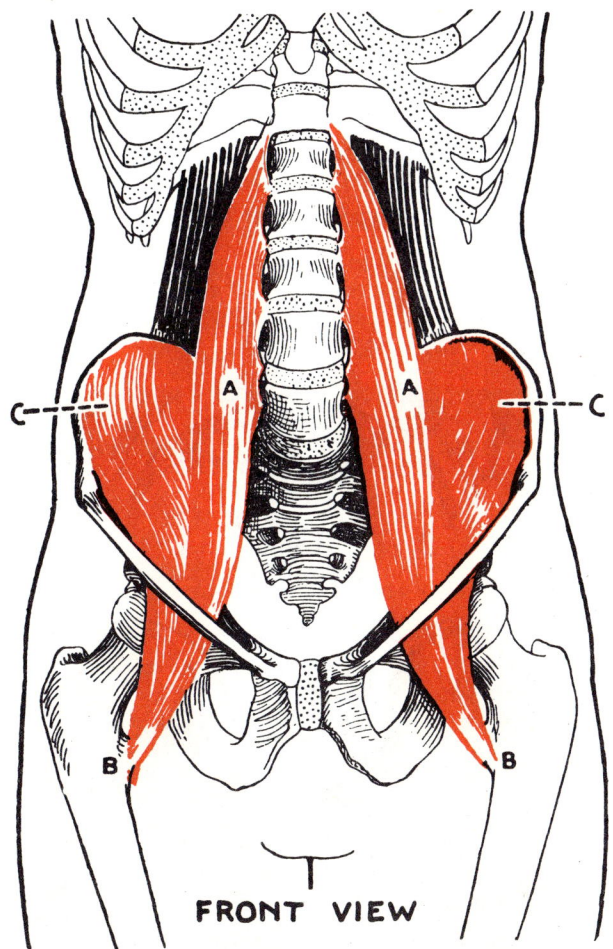

FIGURE 79—The psoas and iliacus muscles

    A—Psoas major
    B—Insertion of psoas and iliacus
        into lesser trochanter
    C—Iliacus

Origin: from the transverse processes and bodies of the last dorsal and all the lumbar vertebrae.

Insertion: into the lesser trochanter below the neck of the femur.

Action: flexes the thigh and assists in internally rotating the femur. When the thigh is fixed it pulls the trunk forward or prevents it falling backward; it assists in maintaining the erect posture.

  (ii) The *iliacus* (the muscle of the ilium. Figure 79) is a broad flat muscle lying on the inner surface of the ilium.

Origin: from the whole inner surface of the ilium.

Insertion: into the lesser trochanter in conjunction with the tendon of the insertion of the psoas.

Action: it has a similar action to that of the psoas.

2. Muscles of the Buttocks

(i) The *gluteus maximus* (the largest muscle of the buttock. Figure 80) is a very large and powerful muscle which gives the buttock its rounded appearance.

Origin: from the posterior portion of the ilium and the back of the sacrum and coccyx.

Insertion: into the posterior aspect of the upper third of the femur below the greater trochanter.

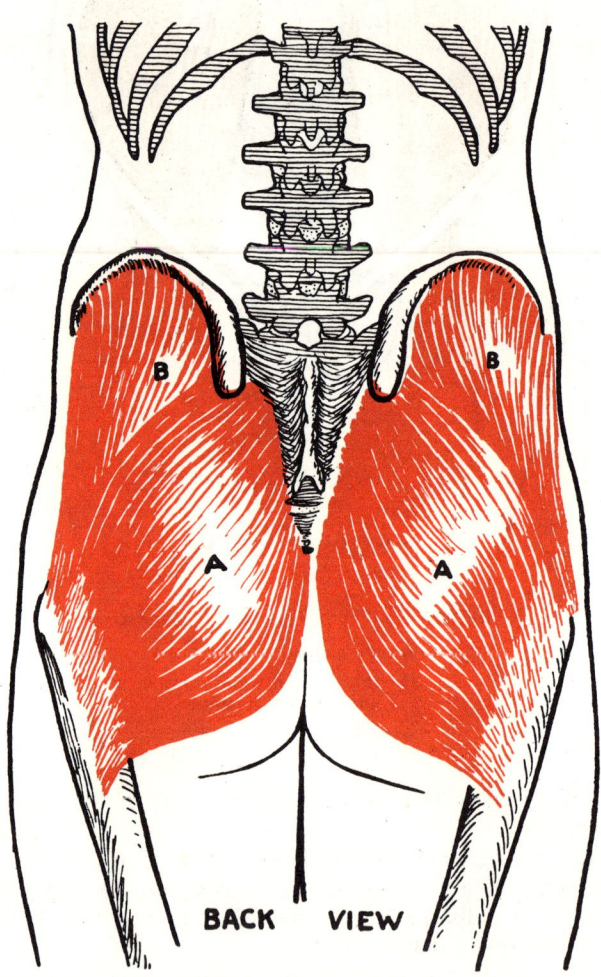

FIGURE 80—The gluteus maximus and medius muscles
A—Gluteus maximus
B—Gluteus medius

Action: extension of the hip joint; it is one of the most important of the muscles which maintain the erect posture and is also the chief muscle of forward propulsion; long distance runners always have well developed glutaeal muscles.

(ii) The *gluteus medius* (Figure 80) and *gluteus minimus* (the medium-sized and smallest muscles of the buttock): these muscles are situated in front of the gluteus maximus; the gluteus medius covers the minimus and the latter cannot therefore be seen in Figure 80.

Origins: from the outer surface of the ilium.

Insertions: into the greater trochanter of the femur.

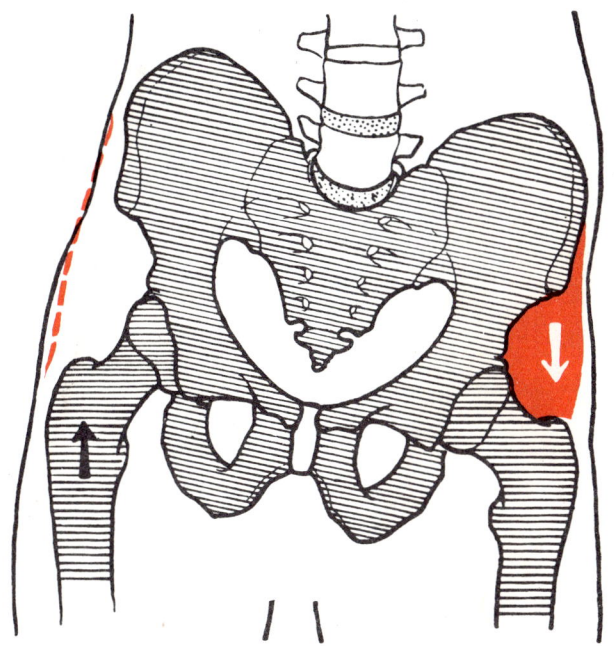

FIGURE 81—The left gluteus medius and minimus tilting the pelvis

Actions: abduction of the femur when the pelvis is the fixed point; if the femur is the fixed point, they tilt the pelvis toward their own side (Figure 81) thus raising the opposite limb from the ground; this action occurs in walking and running. If these muscles are affected so that they cannot perform this action, the gait becomes an exaggerated waddle, like the progression of a duck; the tilting of the pelvis must then be effected by bending the whole trunk sideways from the limb which is being lifted forward.

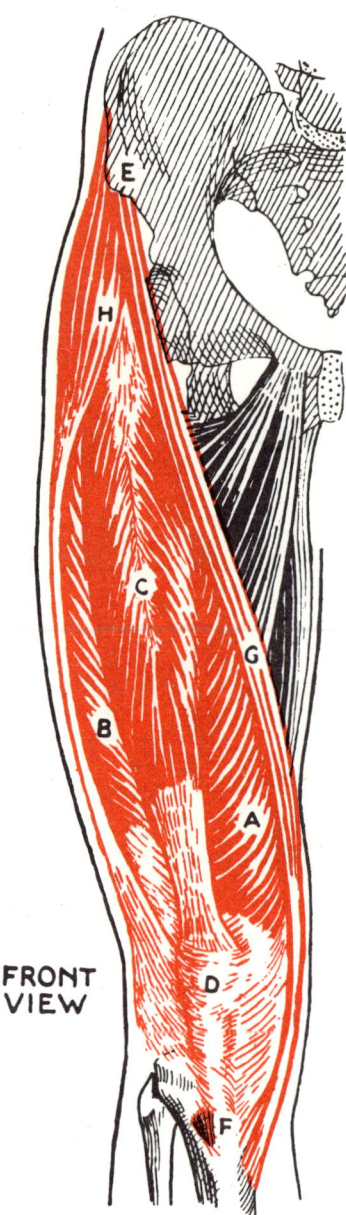

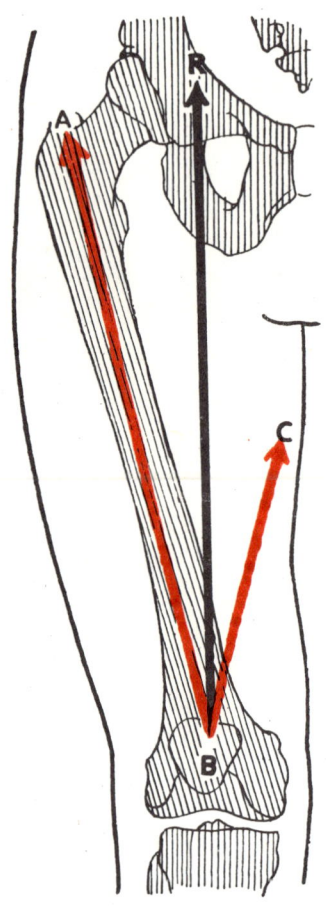

Figure 82—Anterior muscles of the thigh

    A—Inner head of quadriceps
    B—Outer head of quadriceps
    C—Rectus femoris
    D—Patella (enclosed in tendon)
    E—Anterior portion of ilium
    F—Upper end of tibia
    G—Sartorius
    H—Tensor of the broad fascia

Figure 83—Diagram showing resultant direction of pull on the patella

BA—Direction of pull of rectus femoris and the outer and intermediate heads of quadriceps

BC—Direction of pull of the inner head of quadriceps

BR—Direction of the resultant pull

B—Patella

3. Muscles of the Thigh

Anterior group

(i) The *quadriceps* (the four-headed muscle. Figure 82) is a very large and powerful muscle occupying most of the front of the thigh; it has four divisions or *heads*, an inner, an outer, an intermediate and a fourth head, called the rectus femoris (the straight muscle of the thigh). In Figure 82 the intermediate head cannot be seen as it is overlapped by the outer head. The fibres of all four muscles converge towards the patella.

Origin: the inner, outer and intermediate heads arise from the front and sides of the shaft of the femur; the rectus femoris arises from the anterior portion of the ilium.

Insertion: all four heads converge into a single tendon which after enveloping the patella is inserted into a bony prominence on the front of the upper end of the tibia.

Action: extension of the leg upon the thigh: the rectus femoris assists in flexion of the thigh at the hip joint. The quadriceps is a most important muscle of posture.

It may be noticed in Figure 82 that the fleshy part of the inner head of the quadriceps extends almost to the level of the knee joint and that its fibres are directed downward and outward. The reason for this arrangement is that as the pull of the other three heads of the quadriceps is approximately along the line of the femur, BA in Figure 83, and if the outward component of this pull were not counteracted in some way, the patella would dislocate outward; the internal head, however, pulls on the patella along the line BC and the resultant force of the whole muscle group is directed along the line BR, thus keeping the patella in the correct line of movement.

The inner head of the quadriceps is mainly responsible for moving the knee through the last 20 or 30 degrees of extension and when full extension has been reached, it keeps the knee braced back. For this reason, when injuries of the knee which limit extension have occurred, it is usually the first part of the quadriceps to become wasted; its strength, therefore, is an index of the degree of recovery of the injury to the knee.

In cases where one or more ligaments of the knee have been completely ruptured, it is absolutely essential to maintain the power of the quadriceps and particularly of the inner head by appropriate exercises; if this is done conscientiously the instability of the joint may be largely overcome. There are many men with ruptured cruciate ligaments who can still play vigorous football and indulge in other strenuous forms of sport, because they have been properly instructed in maintaining a powerful quadriceps, which can control any laxity of the knee joint almost as efficiently as the ligaments themselves.

(ii) The *sartorius** (Figure 82) is the longest voluntary muscle in the body; it is narrow and rather like a strap.

Origin: from the front of the ilium.

Insertion: into the inner aspect of the upper end of the tibia.

Action: it flexes the thigh on the pelvis and the leg on the thigh; it also rotates the thigh outward and adducts it.

(iii) The *tensor fasciae latae* (Figure 82) is the muscle which tightens the broad tendinous sheet or *fascia* on the outer side of the thigh. It arises from the anterior portion of the crest of the ilium and is inserted into the fascia on the outer side of the leg.

Action: it tightens the fascia and, continuing this action, abducts the thigh. In the erect posture it steadies the pelvis on the thigh and the thigh on the leg.

*This muscle is the tailor's muscle, so called because each brings the lower limb into the crossed leg sitting position.

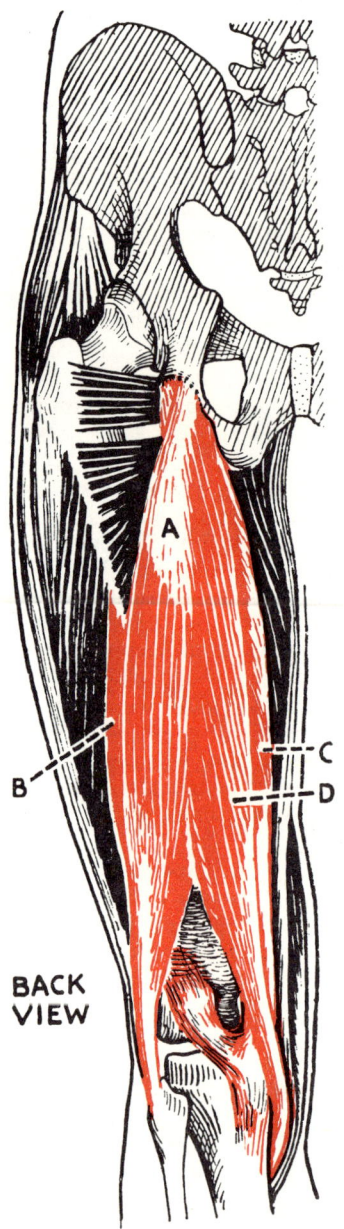
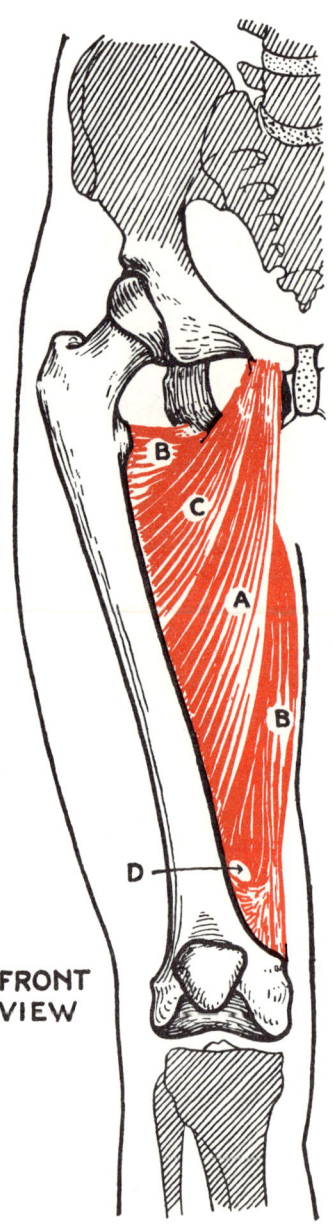

FIGURE 84—The left biceps femoris, semimembranosus and semitendinosus

A—Long head of biceps femoris
B—Short head of biceps femoris
C—Semimembranosus
D—Semitendinosus

FIGURE 85—The right adductor longus, magnus and brevis

A—Adductor longus
B—Adductor magnus
C—Adductor brevis
D—Opening for main blood vessels

Posterior Group

(i) The *biceps femoris* (the two-headed muscle of the thigh. Figure 84) occupies the outer portion of the back of the thigh.

Origin: the long head of the ischium* and the short head from the upper part of the back of the femur.

Insertion: into the upper end of the fibula by a tendon, commonly known as a hamstring.

Action: this muscle is a very powerful flexor of the knee joint. With the legs fixed, each muscle draws the trunk backward as in rising from a stooping position; it plays an important part in maintaining the erect posture.

(ii) The *semimembranosus* and *semitendinosus* (Figure 84) are situated on the inner side of the back of the thigh.

Origins: from the ischium.

Insertions: into the inner aspects of the upper end of the tibia by strong tendons; these are the inner hamstrings.

Actions: like that of the biceps femoris.

Internal group

The *adductor longus*, *adductor magnus* and *adductor brevis* (the long, the large and the short adductors. Figure 85): these three muscles lie one upon the other at the inner side of the thigh; together they form a thick sheet, the shape of a half-haddock.

Origins: from the pubis and ischium.

Insertions: into the posterior aspect of the shaft of the femur; the adductor magnus extends above and below the insertions of the other two muscles.

Actions: adduction of the thigh on the pelvis. They also assist in flexion of the thigh. The fibres of the adductor magnus which arise from the ischium extend the thigh on the pelvis.

The adductor muscles are used more than any other muscle group in riding, the sides of the saddle being grasped between the knees by their contraction.

---

*The *pubis* is that part of the innominate bone below and in front of the acetabulum (the socket for the head of the femur); the *ischium* is that part below and behind the acetabulum.

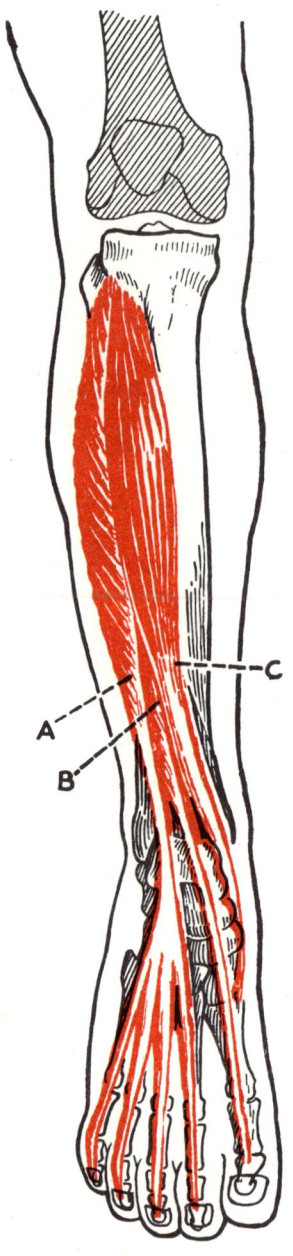

FRONT VIEW

FIGURE 86—The long extensors of the toes and the anterior tibial muscle (right leg)

    A—Long extensor of lesser toes
    B—Long extensor of big toe
    C—Anterior tibial muscle

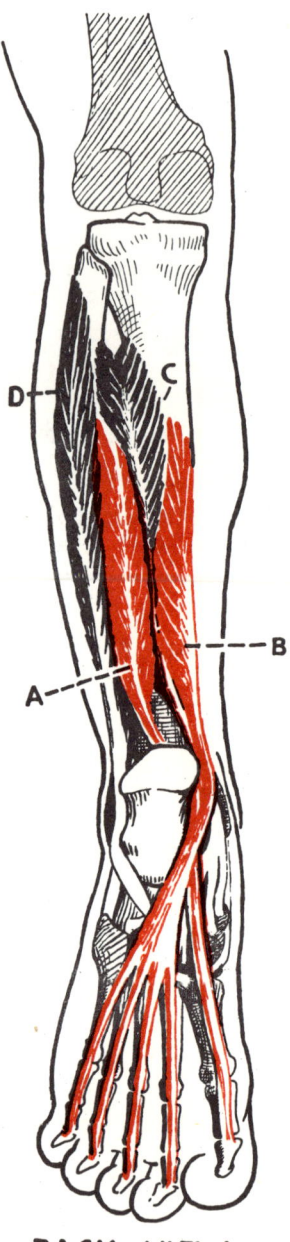

BACK VIEW

FIGURE 87—Posterior muscles of the left leg

    A—Long flexor of big toe
    B—Long flexor of lesser toes
    C—Posterior tibial muscle
    D—Peroneus longus

4. Muscles of the Leg

Anterior group

(i) The *long extensors of the toes* (Figure 86) consist of two muscles, one of which extends the big toe and the other the four lesser toes.

Origins: mainly from the anterior surface of the shaft of the fibula.

Insertions: each muscle becomes tendinous just above the ankle; the tendons pass in front of the ankle joint and across the foot, one being inserted into the last phalanx of the big toe, and the other splitting into four divisions, which are inserted into the last two phalanges of the corresponding toes. As the tendons cross the ankle joint, they are held in position by fibrous ligaments, and to prevent friction against these ligaments, the tendons are enclosed in special tendon sheaths which contain a lubricating fluid.

Actions: extension of the toes; both muscles also assist in dorsiflexing the foot.

(ii) The *anterior tibial* muscle (Figure 86) lies mainly over the tibia; it can be felt lying along the sharp edge of that bone.

Origin: from the shaft of the tibia.

Insertion: its tendon passes over the front of the ankle joint to be inserted into the first cuneiform and first metatarsal bones on the inner border of the foot.

Action: dorsiflexion of the foot; it is also a strong invertor of the foot and supports the inner border of the longitudinal arch.

Posterior group

(i) The *long flexors of the toes* (Figure 87): these two muscles lie on the posterior surfaces of the tibia and fibula.

Origins: from the posterior surfaces of the tibia and fibula.

Insertions: the tendons pass round the inner side of the ankle and under the foot; one tendon is inserted into the phalanx of the big toe, the other splits into four divisions which are inserted into the last phalanges of the corresponding toes.

Actions: in addition to flexing the toes they assist in plantar flexion of the foot.

(ii) The *posterior tibial* muscle (Figures 87 and 88) is an important muscle situated between the tibia and fibula at the back of the leg.

Origin: from the posterior surfaces of the tibia and fibula.

Insertion: its tendon passes with the long flexor tendons round the inner side of the ankle joint and is inserted into every bone of the tarsus, except the talus, and into the bases of the middle three metatarsals.

Action: its chief action is plantar flexion, but it is also a strong invertor of the foot. By means of its broad insertion it acts as the main support of the inner side of the longitudinal arch of the foot.

(iii) The *gastrocnemius* (the belly-shaped muscle of the leg. Figure 89) and the *soleus* (the muscle shaped like the sole fish. Figure 89) together form the calf muscles. The soleus covers the long flexor and posterior tibial muscles and is itself almost covered by the gastrocnemius.

Origins: the gastrocnemius arises by two separate attachments, one to each of the condyles of the femur; the soleus arises from the posterior surfaces of the upper ends of the tibia and fibula.

Insertions: the tendons of the two muscles blend into one to form the well known Achilles tendon which is inserted into the back of the calcaneus. The Achilles tendon is the strongest and thickest in the body. This fact must have been well known to Thetis, the mother of Achilles, when she gripped him by this tendon to dip him in the waters of the Styx.

Actions: mainly plantar flexion; this is usually performed with the foot as fixed point, thus raising the body on the toes; the gastrocnemius, by reason of its attachment above the knee joint, assists in flexing the knee joint.

These two muscles provide the normal spring to the gait; they are the chief jumping muscles.

External group

The *peroneus longus* (Figures 87 and 88) and *peroneus brevis* (the long and short muscles of the brooch bone or fibula): both muscles are situated on the outer side of the leg.

Origins: from the outer side of the fibula.

Insertions: the tendon of the peroneus longus crosses underneath the longitudinal arch of the foot to be inserted into the base of the first metatarsal and into the adjoining cuneiform bone. Thus with the tendon of the posterior tibial muscle it forms a sling which supports the crown of the longitudinal arch (Figure 88).

The peroneus brevis is inserted into the base of the fifth metatarsal.

Actions: both muscles act as evertors of the foot.

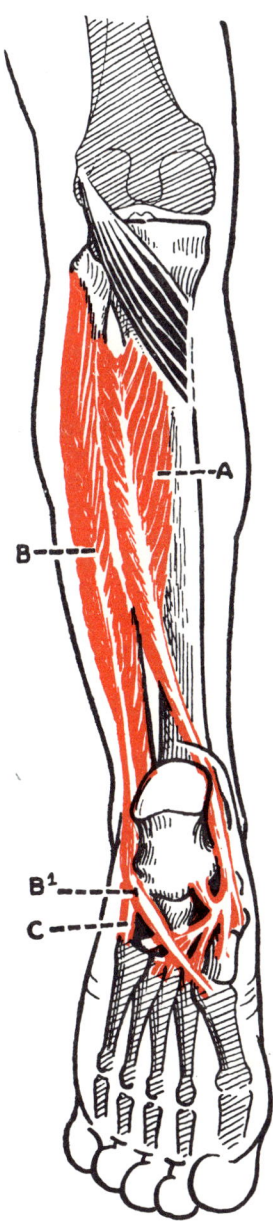

BACK VIEW

FIGURE 88—Showing insertion of the left posterior tibial muscle into the bones of the foot (viewed from below)

A—Posterior tibial muscle
B—Peroneus longus
B¹—Tendon of Peroneus longus
C—Tendon of peroneus brevis

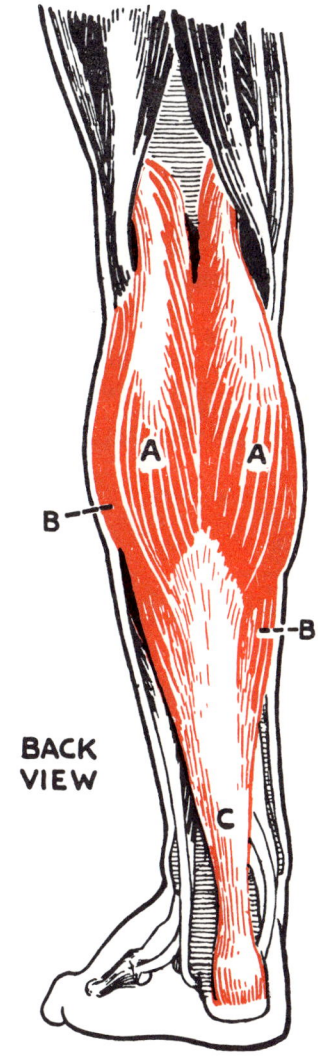

FIGURE 89—The calf muscles of the left leg

A—Gastrocnemius
B—Soleus (outer and inner edges only are visible)
C—Achilles tendon

5. Muscles of the Foot

The four layers of small muscles in the foot are covered by a very strong and broad tendinous sheet (Figure 90) which acts as the tie-beam to the arch of the foot.

The muscles, with very few exceptions, run parallel to the longitudinal arch, because their main function is to pull on its two pillars and thus prevent it flattening.

The arch of the foot is primarily maintained by muscular support and secondarily by ligaments. As mentioned above the peroneus longus and posterior tibial muscle support the crown of the arch by a sling-like arrangement; the small muscles maintain the pillars in their correct position. The ligaments give additional support, but soon become stretched if they are subjected to prolonged strains. A flat foot, that is one in which the longitudinal arch has flattened, need not necessarily give rise to pain; the presence of pain depends on the state of the small muscles; for example, most ballet dancers have flat feet, but very strong foot muscles and supple joints of the tarsus; this type of flat foot is not accompanied by any disability or pain; but the flat foot in which the muscles are weak usually has stiff tarsal joints and the condition becomes painful, because, the muscles being too weak to do their normal share of work, the whole body weight is thrown on the ligaments; if this goes on for long periods the ligaments become slightly inflamed and painful adhesions* start to form around them and the foot becomes gradually stiffer. This results in postural defects and difficulty in walking, because the foot is no longer sufficiently flexible to make delicate adjustments of balance.

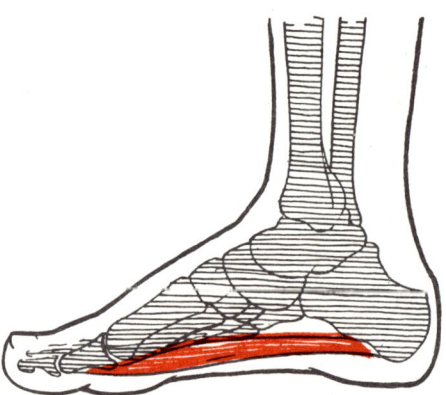

FIGURE 90—Showing the tendinous sheet on the sole of the foot acting as tie-beam to the longitudinal arch

---

*An adhesion is scar tissue which forms as a result of the healing of some local inflammation; scar tissue contracts as it heals, binding together the surrounding structures, and may thus cause pain.

SUMMARY OF MUSCLE ACTIONS

The names of the various muscles which co-operate with one another to produce movement at certain joints are named below; the muscles are mentioned in the order of their importance in the particular movement described.

1. Movements of the Cervical Part of the Vertebral Column

(i) Flexion: the sternomastoids, longi colli and scaleni.

(ii) Extension: the splenii capitis, splenii cervicis, trapezii and upper part of the long muscles of the spine.

(iii) Lateral flexion: the sternomastoid, scaleni, levator scapulae, trapezius and upper part of long spinal muscles all of one side.

(iv) Rotation: the sternomastoid of one side, the small rotators of the cervical part of the vertebral column and the upper part of the long spinal muscles.

2. Respiration

(i) Quiet respiration: the diaphragm, recti abdominis, oblique and transverse muscles and the intercostals.

(ii) Deep respiration: all the muscles under (i), assisted by the sternomastoid, scaleni, pectorals, latissimus dorsi and quadratus lumborum of both sides.

3. Movements of the Dorsal and Lumbar parts of Vertebral Column

(i) Flexion: the recti abdominis, oblique muscles of the abdomen and psoas and iliacus of both sides. Gravity performs most of this action in the erect position.

(ii) Extension: the long spinal muscles. The latissimus dorsi and trapezius of both sides can assist this movement when the shoulder girdle is fixed.

(iii) Lateral flexion: the oblique muscles, rectus abdominis, spinal muscles, latissimus dorsi, quadratus lumborum and psoas, all of one side.

(iv) Rotation: the external oblique of one side with the internal oblique of the opposite side assisted by the long and short spinal muscles.

4. Movements of the Shoulder Girdle*

(i) Backward rotation or bracing the shoulders back; the trapezius, rhomboideus major and rhomboideus minor.

(ii) Forward rotation: the serratus anterior, pectoralis major and pectoralis minor.

(iii) Elevation or shrugging the shoulders; the trapezius and levator scapulae.

(iv) Depression; latissimus dorsi and lower fibres of the trapezius.

5. Movements at the Shoulder Joint

(i) Flexion or forward elevation of the upper arm; the pectoralis major (clavicular portion), the anterior fibres of the deltoid, the biceps and the coracobrachialis.

(ii) Extension: the posterior fibres of the deltoid, the latissimus dorsi, the long head of triceps and the teres major.

(iii) Abduction (Figure 93): through the first 10 or 15 degrees, the deltoid assisted by the supraspinatus; from 15 to approximately 90 degrees, the deltoid alone; from 90 to 145 degrees, the serratus anterior with the trapezius assisting and controlling rotation of the scapula while the deltoid, supraspinatus and small muscles of the shoulder keep the shoulder joint fixed. At this point the humerus must be externally rotated, if that has not already been done, in order to raise the arm vertically above the head. This final movement is completed by the deltoid, mainly by its anterior fibres.

*The movements described refer to one half of the shoulder girdle.

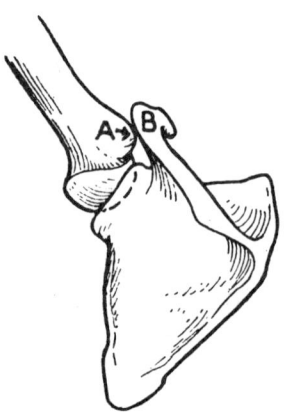

FIGURE 91—Amount of abduction possible without external rotation of arm
A—Greater tuberosity impinging on acromion (B)

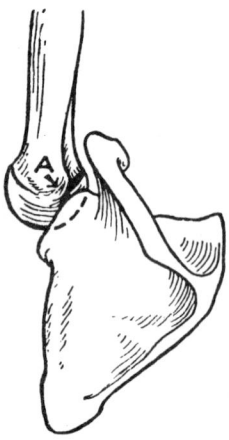

FIGURE 92—Amount of abduction possible with external rotation of arm
A—Greater tuberosity facing backward, allowing movement of abduction to continue

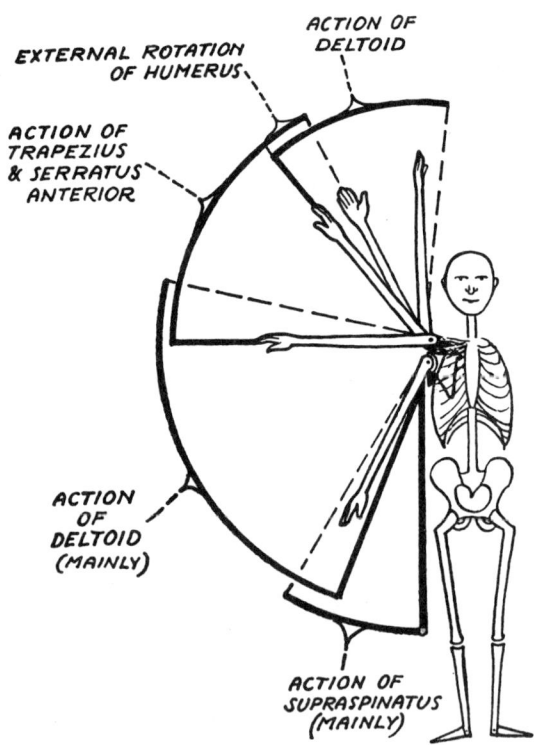

FIGURE 93—Diagram showing the approximate range of action of the muscles which perform abduction of the shoulder

(iv) Adduction: the pectoralis major, latissimus dorsi, infraspinatus, teres major and minor, subscapularis and long head of triceps.

(v) External rotation: the infraspinatus and teres minor.

(vi) Internal rotation: the pectoralis major (sternal portion), subscapularis, latissimus dorsi and teres major.

6. Movements at the Elbow Joint

(i) Flexion: the brachialis, biceps brachialis, brachioradialis, and the flexor group of the forearm muscles.

(ii) Extension: the triceps.

7. Movements of the Forearm

(i) Pronation: the pronator teres and pronator quadratus.

(ii) Supination: the biceps and short supinator muscle.

8. Movements at the Wrist

(i) Palmar flexion: the flexors of the wrist and the long flexors of the fingers and thumb.

(ii) Dorsiflexion: the extensors of the wrist and the long extensors of the fingers and thumb.

(iii) Radial deviation: the flexor and extensor of the wrist, which are inserted on the radial side of the carpus, and the long abductor and extensors of the thumb.

(iv) Ulnar deviation: the flexor and extensor of the wrist which are inserted into the ulnar side of the carpus.

9. Movements at the Hip Joint

(i) Flexion: the rectus femoris (of the quadriceps), psoas, iliacus, sartorius, and adductores.

(ii) Extension: the gluteus maximus, biceps femoris, semimembranosus, semitendinosus and the fibres of the adductor magnus which arise from the ischium.

(iii) Abduction: the gluteus medius, gluteus minimus, sartorius and tensor fasciae latae.

(iv) External rotation: the small muscles arising from the hip bone and inserted into the back of the upper end of the femur; also the sartorius.

(v) Internal rotation: the gluteus medius, gluteus minimus, tensor fasciae latae and psoas.

10. Movements at the Knee Joint

(i) Flexion: the biceps femoris, semimembranosus, semitendinosus, sartorius and gastrocnemius.

(ii) Extension: the quadriceps.

11. Movements at the Ankle Joint

(i) Dorsiflexion: the anterior tibial muscle and long extensors of the toes.

(ii) Plantar flexion: the gastocnemius, soleus, posterior tibial muscle and long flexors of the toes.

12. Movements at the Joints between the Talus and Calcaneus and the Talus and the Navicular Bone

(i) Inversion: the posterior tibial and anterior tibial muscles.

(ii) Eversion: the peroneus longus and peroneus brevis.

ILLUSTRATIONS OF THE SUPERFICIAL MUSCLES

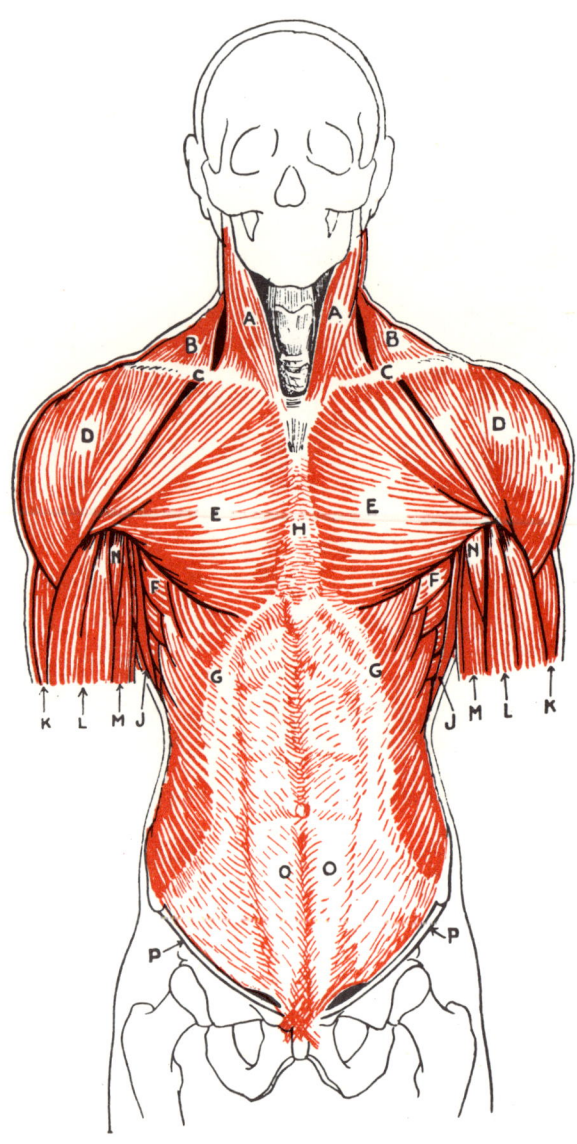

FIGURE 94—The muscles of the trunk and shoulder girdle viewed from the front

A—Sternomastoid
B—Trapezius
C—Clavicle
D—Deltoid
E—Pectoralis major
F—Serratus anterior
G—External oblique
H—Sternum
J—Latissimus dorsi
K—Brachialis
L—Biceps brachialis
M—Triceps (long head)
N—Coracobrachialis
O—Rectus abdominis covered by aponeurosis
P—Inguinal ligament

85

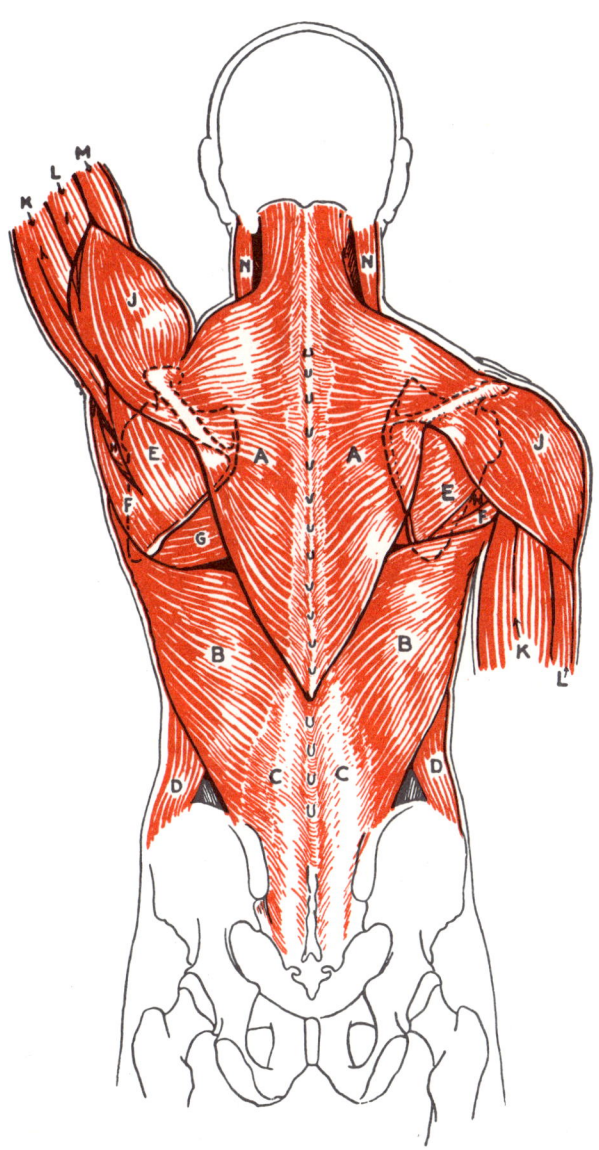

FIGURE 95—The muscles of the trunk and shoulder girdle viewed from behind

A—Trapezius
B—Latissimus dorsi
C—Prominence due to underlying sacrospinalis
D—External oblique
E—Infraspinatus
F—Teres major
G—Rhomboideus major
H—Teres minor
J—Deltoid
K—Triceps
L—Brachialis
M—Biceps brachialis
N—Sternomastoid

(In the living body with the left arm raised the left scapula will be approximately one inch higher than shown in the diagram)

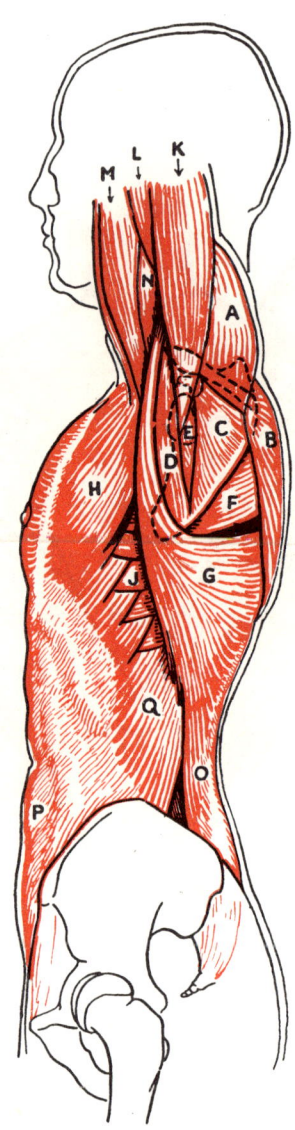

FIGURE 96—The muscles of the trunk and shoulder girdle viewed from the side

A—Deltoid
B—Trapezius
C—Infraspinatus
D—Teres major
E—Teres minor
F—Rhomboideus major
G—Latissimus dorsi
H—Pectoralis major
J—Serratus anterior
K—Triceps (long head)
L—Brachialis
M—Biceps brachialis
N—Coracobrachialis
O—Latissimus dorsi
P—Rectus abdominis
Q—External oblique

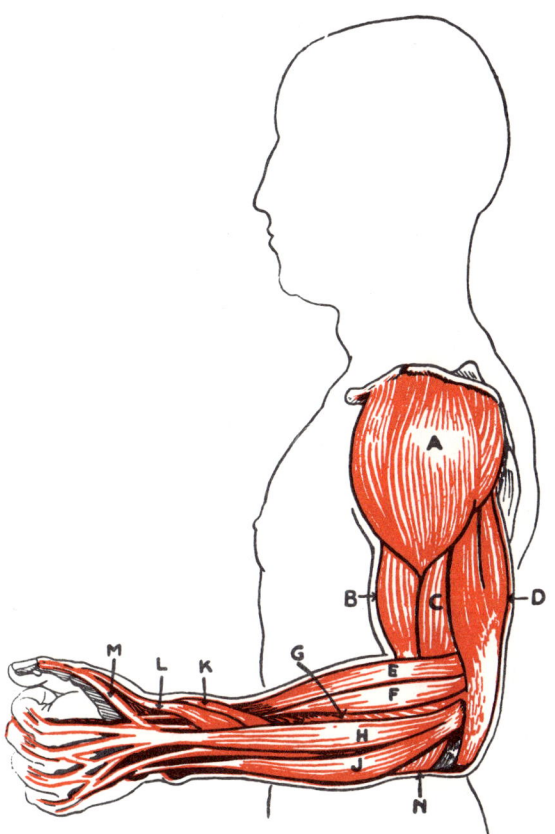

FIGURE 97—The muscles of the arm and forearm viewed from the side

A—Deltoid
B—Biceps brachialis
C—Brachialis
D—Triceps
E—Brachioradialis
F and G—Extensors of the wrist
H—Long extensor of the fingers
J—Extensor of the wrist
K—Long abductor of the thumb
L—Short extensor of the thumb
M—Long extensor of the thumb
N—Anconaeus

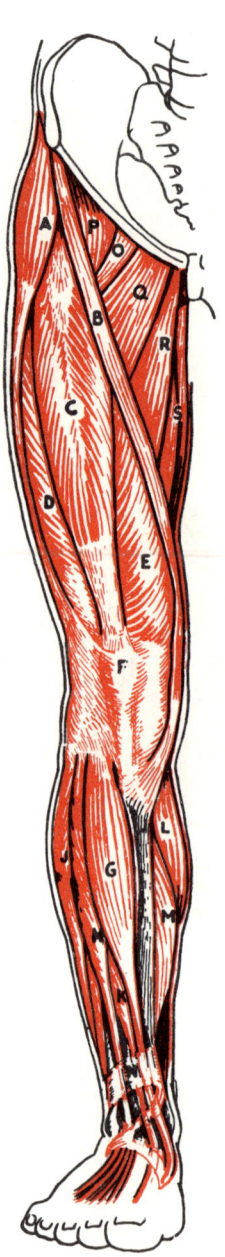

A—Tensor fasciae latae
B—Sartorius
C—Rectus femoris of quadriceps
D—Outer head of quadriceps
E—Inner head of quadriceps
F—Patella
G—Anterior tibial muscle
H—Long extensor of the toes
J—Peroneus longus
K—Long extensor of big toe
L—Inner edge of gastrocnemius
M—Inner edge of soleus
N—Ligament maintaining extensor tendons in position
O—Psoas
P—Iliacus
Q—Pectineus
R—Adductor longus
S—Adductor magnus

FIGURE 98—The muscles of the thigh and leg viewed from the front

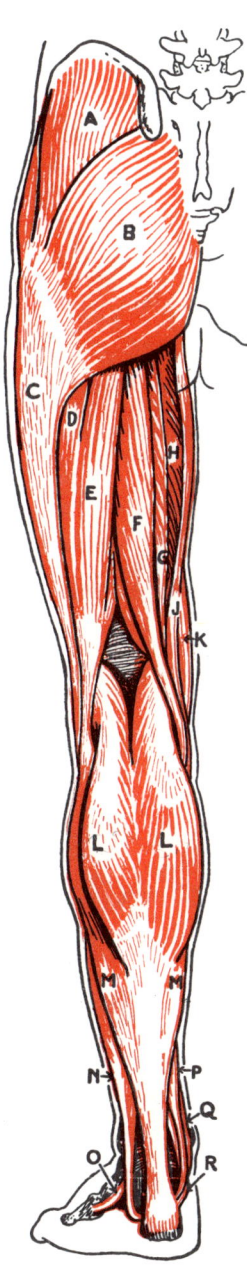

A—Gluteus medis
B—Gluteus maximus
C—Broad fascia of the thigh
D—Short head of biceps femoris
E—Long head of biceps femoris
F—Semitendinosus
G—Semimembranosus
H—Adductor magnus
J—Gracilis
K—Sartorius
L—Gastrocnemius
M—Soleus
N—Peroneus longus
O—Peroneus brevis
P—Long flexor of the toes
Q—Posterior tibial muscle
R—Long flexor of the big toe

FIGURE 99—The muscles of the thigh and leg viewed from behind

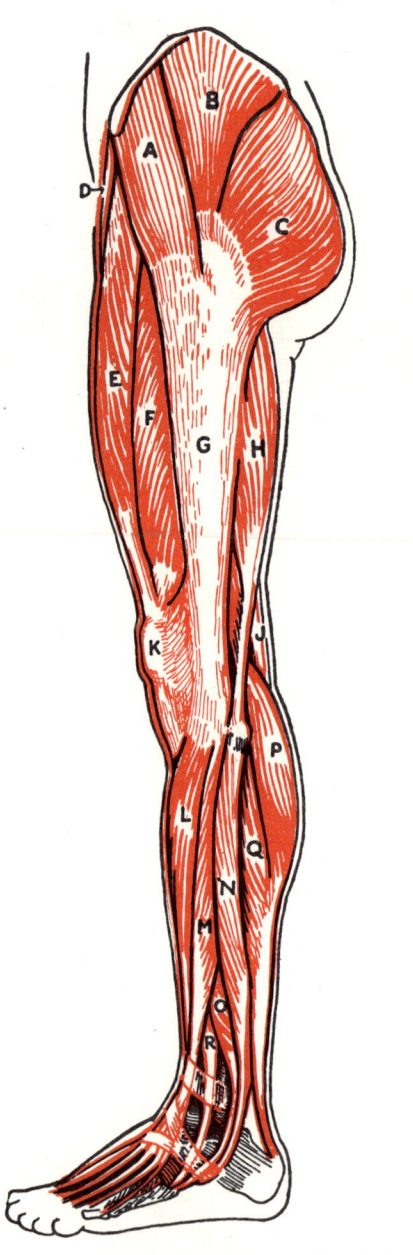

A—Tensor fasciae latae
B—Gluteus medius
C—Gluteus maximus
D—Sartorius
E—Rectus femoris of quadriceps
F—Outer head of quadriceps
G—Broad fascia of the thigh
H—Long head of biceps
J—Semitendinosus
K—Patella
L—Anterior tibial muscle
M—Long extensor of the toes
N—Peroneus longus
O—Peroneus brevis
P—Gastrocnemius
Q—Soleus
R—Peroneus tertius

FIGURE 100—The muscles of the thigh and leg viewed from the side

CHAPTER II
PHYSIOLOGY
SECTION 1—THE VASCULAR SYSTEM

The Blood

Blood is the fluid medium by means of which every structure in the body is nourished; it is moved or circulated through the various systems of the body by the pumping action of the heart. The blood conveys oxygen and certain products of digestion to the tissues which require them; it also takes away from the tissues the waste products which accumulate, for example, after severe muscular activity and conveys them to the excretory organs of the body.

Blood also provides the tissues with a mobile defence against the invasion of bacteria, for it contains certain cells which congregate round the area in which the invading bacteria are attempting to establish themselves; as soon as these cells have successfully surrounded and sealed off the invaders, they attack and destroy them.

The Composition of Blood

Blood is a fluid, mobile type of body tissue. To the naked eye it appears to be nothing more than a red fluid, but if a drop of fresh blood is examined under a microscope, many hundreds of small red cells, the *red blood corpuscles*, can be seen suspended in a pale yellow fluid called the *plasma*; there are other cells present which cannot be distinguished without special staining;* these are the *white corpuscles* which are the bacterial scavengers; they are not nearly as numerous as the red blood corpuscles. The plasma and the cells which it contains make up about an eleventh part of the total body weight of the normal adult. The average volume of blood is about six litres or ten and a half pints.

The *plasma* is a fluid consisting of water, proteins† and certain mineral salts of which ordinary salt, *sodium chloride*, is the chief. The proteins include a substance which is responsible for the clotting of blood.

The *red blood corpuscles* are circular biconcave discs (Figure 101); each consists of a fine membrane containing a thick red liquid. The redness of the liquid is due to a pigment called *haemoglobin*.

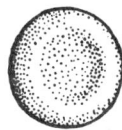 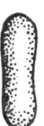

FIGURE 101—Surface and profile view of a red blood corpuscle. (Magnified about 1,500 times)

The chief property of haemoglobin is its power of carrying oxygen from surroundings where oxygen is plentiful to those where it is not. In the presence of an abundance of oxygen, for example in the air of the lungs, haemoglobin absorbs oxygen, to release it later in the tissues of the body where all available oxygen is being used and is in consequence present in small quantities only. Blood which contains much oxygen is bright red in colour, whereas that which has only a little is dull red. This may be illustrated when blood is withdrawn from a vein; it is dull red because it has given up its oxygen to the tissues but if it is shaken in a test tube, mixing it freely with the oxygen in the air, it, becomes bright red.

The red blood corpuscles are formed mainly in the bone marrow. In the healthy adult there are five to six million of them per cubic millimetre of blood. Anaemia is a condition in which there is a shortage of haemoglobin, usually accompanied by a fall in the number of red blood corpuscles.

* The individual characteristics of various tissues in the body may be more clearly distinguished under the microscope when the tissues have been stained with certain dyes.

† A protein is a complex chemical compound, made up mainly of nitrogen, carbon, hydrogen and oxygen.

The *white cells* are generally larger than the red cells; they are circular, but unlike the red cells contain a special body within the cell called a nucleus.*
There are several types of white cells, but their functions are much the same, namely the sealing off of infection from the blood stream and the destruction of bacteria within the tissues and the blood stream. Some are formed in the bone marrow and others in the *lymphatic* glands, which are small rounded lumps of glandular tissue distributed throughout the body; as is well known, these glands swell and become painful when any local infection is present.

The Circulation (Figure 102)

The heart distributes blood to the various parts of the body through a system of tubes; those which convey the blood away from the heart are called *arteries* and those which bring it to the heart are termed *veins*.

The arteries are constructed of involuntary muscle and elastic tissue, and are capable of withstanding considerable pressure from within. Near the heart they are about one inch in diameter; they decrease gradually in size as they give off more and more branches. When they have reached the tissue which they supply, they break up into a fine network of small tubes called *capillaries* which may be so small that the red blood corpuscles have to pass through them in single file. The capillary walls are very thin and allow an exchange of fluids and gases between the red cells and the surrounding tissues. Each capillary has two ends, an arterial end which is the termination of the artery, and a venous end which is the beginning of the vein. The venous capillaries merge to form small veins which gradually get bigger as they receive more tributaries on their way back to the heart. Veins have thinner walls than arteries and less elastic tissue, because they are not subjected to so much pressure from within; they contain muscle fibres in their walls.

All veins containing blood which has to flow against gravity are provided with sets of valves at varying intervals along their course; these valves allow the blood to flow in the direction of the heart, but prevent it flowing in the reverse direction under the force of gravity. If it were not for the presence of valves the venous blood flow in the lower limbs would be working against the gravitational weight of a column of blood extending up to the heart; but by means of valves this weight is split up, so that it becomes no more than the weight of a column of blood extending between one set of valves and another. An injury to one of these sets of valves may be followed by the appearance of varicose veins.

The Heart (Figure 103)

The heart is the central organ of the circulatory system; it maintains the pressure of the circulation and controls the rate of flow through the system. It receives blood from the veins at a low pressure and pumps it into the blood vessels of the lungs for oxygenation. The blood flowing back from the lungs is again received by the heart and pumped into the arteries which branch out to all parts of the body.

The heart therefore maintains two systems of circulation of the blood; one through the lungs and the other through all the other parts of the body. For this reason the heart is divided into two sections which do not communicate one with the other. These sections are known as the right side and the left sides of the heart. The right side receives the impure blood from the great veins which have collected it from the general or *systemic* circulation and pumps it through the lungs for re-oxygenation; the left side receives the oxygenated blood which has passed through the lung or *pulmonary* circulation and pumps it into the arteries of the systemic circulation to nourish the tissues.

* The nucleus is the specialised part of a cell which controls its life and growth. It also plays an important part in the formation of new cells. The red blood corpuscles in the blood stream are exceptional in not containing nuclei.

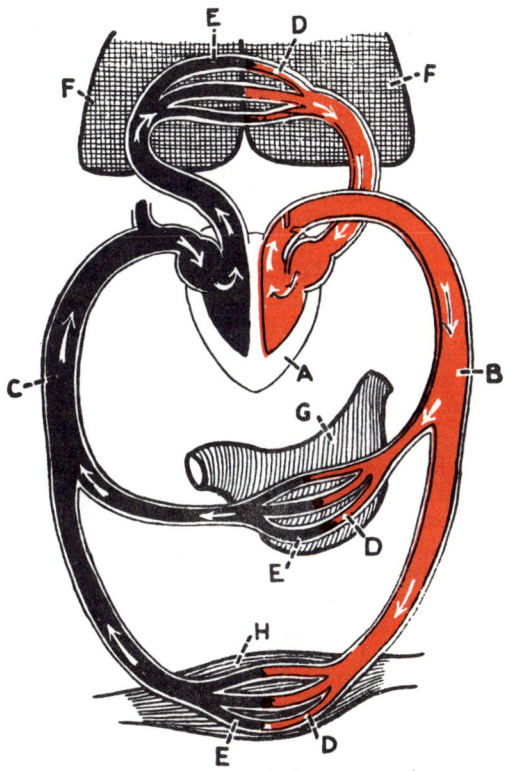

FIGURE 102—Diagram of circulation through the lungs, the stomach and muscle
A—Heart
B—Main artery (aorta)
C—Main vein
D—Arterial end of capillary
E—Venous end of capillary
F—Lungs
G—Stomach
H—Muscle

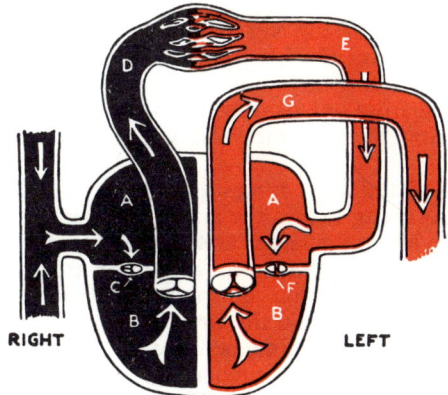

FIGURE 103—Diagram showing circulation of blood through the heart; the blackened portions represent venous blood
A—Auricle
B—Ventricle
C—Tricuspid valve
D—Pulmonary artery
E—Pulmonary vein
F—Bicuspid valve (mitral valves)
G—Main artery of the body or aorta

Structure and Position

The heart is a hollow organ with thick muscular walls; it is situated behind the sternum, a little to the left of the middle line of the body, and the left lung, in order to accommodate it, is notched and rather smaller than the right. Each side of the heart contains two chambers, one called the *auricle* and the other the *ventricle*. Dark blood from the great veins passes through a simple opening into the right auricle and thence is pumped through an opening guarded by a valve, the *tricuspid* valve, into the right ventricle; the right ventricle pumps the blood at pressure into the *pulmonary artery** whence it passes through the lungs where it is oxygenated and becomes bright red in consequence, and into the vein of the lungs or *pulmonary vein*. The pulmonary vein ends without a valve in the left auricle, which pumps blood through an opening guarded by the *bicuspid* valve into the left ventricle. The left ventricle pumps this arterial blood into the main artery of the systemic circulation, the *aorta*, and the blood passes round the body to find its way back into the great veins on the right side of the heart.

Function

The rhythm of the heart is determined by a mechanism, partly nervous and partly muscular, which will not be described in this book. However, the result of the mechanism is that a wave of contraction of the heart muscle is initiated about six times every five seconds, when the body is at rest. This wave of contraction first involves both auricles simultaneously so that they contract, the right forcing venous blood into the right ventricle, and the left forcing oxygenated blood into the left ventricle. Within a very short space of time, about one-eighth of a second, the wave spreads to the ventricles, which contract simultaneously with great force, shutting the tricuspid (right) and bicuspid (left) valves by mechanical action. The blood is thus forced into the pulmonary artery from the right ventricle and the aorta from the left ventricle, and is prevented from running back into the ventricles by the automatic closure of the sets of valves in these arteries owing to the back pressure of blood in them.

These heart valves are apt to be injured by the disease called *rheumatic fever*; they may then become incompetent, which means that they can no longer make a watertight fit. If the valve affected is the tricuspid or the bicuspid, blood rushes back into the right or left auricle when the ventricles contract, or, if the valve is one of those in the pulmonary artery or aorta, the blood rushes back into one or other of the ventricles after their contraction. Another condition which may affect the heart valves after rheumatic fever is *stenosis* or narrowing. It may affect any valve and by causing an obstruction to the normal flow of blood from one chamber to another, it embarrasses the action of the heart. Occasionally the same valve may be both narrowed and incompetent.

Each contraction of the heart forces a quantity of blood into the systemic circulation and in so doing causes the aorta to expand. The extra pressure is conducted as a wave along the larger arteries to all parts of the body and may be felt as the *pulse*. This may be felt in any large artery; the radial artery at the wrist is generally used to take the pulse, because there it runs only just below the surface of the skin and the wrist is a normally exposed part of the body. No pulse can be felt in veins, because the pressure wave has expended itself in the small capillaries of the circulation.

Blood Pressure

It is common knowledge that fluid does not travel along a system of pipes unless it is driven by something which delivers it into the system under pressure The circulation of the blood through a huge number of arteries, capillaries and

---

* The pulmonary artery is the artery of the lungs; it holds blood at pressure and has thick walls of elastic and muscle tissue. However, it contains dark blood, commonly called venous blood, and not bright red blood, commonly called arterial blood.

veins is maintained by a considerable pressure supplied by the contractions of the heart muscle. The pulmonary circulation is smaller in length and volume than the systemic circulation, consequently blood is not delivered into it at such a great pressure as it is into the latter. The pressure in the aorta at rest at the moment of ventricular contraction is approximately equal to that exerted by a column of mercury 180 millimetres in height or a column of water of 7 feet 6 inches. This pressure rapidly falls to about 125 millimetres of mercury in the larger arteries of the head, trunk and limbs. It can be demonstrated with a blood pressure apparatus, usually applied to the upper arm. This apparatus consists of a long rubber bag in a covering of cloth. The rubber bag is connected by tubes to a simple pump and to a glass tube with a small reservoir at its lower end containing mercury. The rubber bag is strapped round the upper arm, fastened and then pumped up until the pulse at the wrist has disappeared. At this point it is evident that the pressure in the bag is equal to the blood pressure in the main artery of the arm, and since the pressure in the bag has pushed up a column of mercury in the glass tube, the length of the column may be read on the scale.

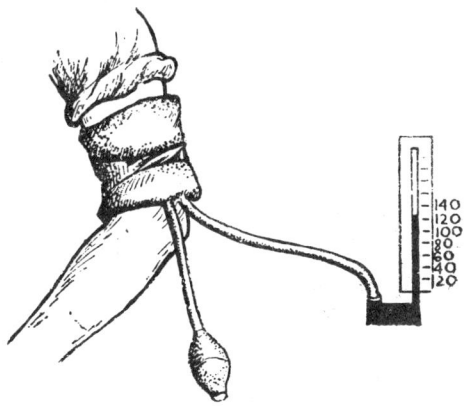

FIGURE 104—Method of measuring blood pressure

The pressure of blood in arteries may also be demonstrated by accident, when an artery is injured; the blood spurts out in a bright red jet which shows a little added pulsation each time the heart beats.

The pressure in the system is largely absorbed by the friction of the blood against the blood vessels, particularly the smallest arteries, so that by the time the blood has reached the veins it is at a pressure of a few millimetres of mercury only; when a vein is cut dull red blood oozes slowly from the wound.

The arterial blood pressure of healthy persons varies according to their activities and age. It is raised during exercise and is low during sleep. It rises as age increases, because the hardening of arteries which accompanies age causes an increase in the resistance to the circulation which makes necessary an increased pressure to maintain it. Young people can tolerate a considerable rise in blood pressure during severe exercise without any damaging after-effects, but older people are running a definite risk of overstraining their circulatory systems, if they attempt to take exercise of a type likely to produce a large rise in blood pressure. When a man reaches middle age he must begin to grade his exercise according to his individual capacity; he must learn his own limitations and not allow himself to reach that stage of over-exertion where he experiences a sense of general bodily discomfort. The truth of this is aptly put in the saying 'a man is as old as his arteries'.

The Rate and Output of the Heart

The oxygen requirements of the body are considerably increased during exercise; the heart is then stimulated by a nervous and chemical mechanism to beat much faster in order to increase the rate of blood flow, and in addition to give a greater output of blood with each contraction. The return of blood to the heart is accelerated by the increased rate of respiration which helps to draw the blood into the great veins near the heart, and also by the increased activity of the muscles which, by their contractions, propel the blood through the veins more quickly. The rate of the heart beat of a man running at nine miles an hour for ten minutes may rise to 140 per minute and the output from a normal 5 litres per minute to as much as 30 litres or 52 pints per minute.

SECTION 2— THE RESPIRATORY SYSTEM

The *respiratory system* consists of the *air passages* and the *lungs*. Its functions are the provision of oxygen for the blood and the removal of certain waste products from the body, the most important of which is carbon dioxide.

The Air Passages

The *air passages* (Figure 105) are the *nasal passages*, the *pharynx* or back of the throat, the *larynx* which contains the vocal chords and lies behind the Adam's apple, the windpipe and the large and small divisions of the bronchial tubes.

The *nasal passages* (Figure 106) play a very important part in respiration, their function in the body can be compared to that of an air conditioning machine which filters and warms the air before it is used.

The nasal cavity is divided into a right and left nasal passage by a partition called the *septum*. On the outer walls of each nasal passage are three bony flanges. On each side there are two *sinuses* or cavities, one in the cheek bone and the other in the forehead bone immediately above the eye; each sinus is connected to the nasal passage of the same side by a small opening The whole surface area of the nasal passages and sinuses is lined by *mucous membrane* which secretes a clear, slightly viscous fluid called mucus. Such a secretion, which is particularly in evidence on very cold days, enables the nasal passages to act as air filters by causing dust particles and bacteria to adhere to the sticky mucous membrane; the secretion itself is able to destroy certain bacteria. A moist mucous membrane is essential to health; when it becomes dry in a hot, stuffy atmosphere its efficiency as a germ trap is at once impaired and infection may gain access to the body; a common cold may be contracted in this way.

The large surface area of mucous membrane covering the bones of the nasal passages is liberally supplied with small blood vessels and the blood in these vessels gives up its heat to warm the air before it reaches the lungs. The air thus warmed passes through the pharynx and into the larynx and thence between the vocal chords into the windpipe; the windpipe divides into two bronchial tubes, one going to each lung. Within the lung tissue each bronchial tube divides many times until its branches become invisible to the naked eye ; these small branches (Figure 107) open into the *air sacs*. The walls of the windpipe and the two large bronchial tubes are composed largely of cartilage which acts as a stiffening material to prevent collapse of the walls and obstruction of the airway.

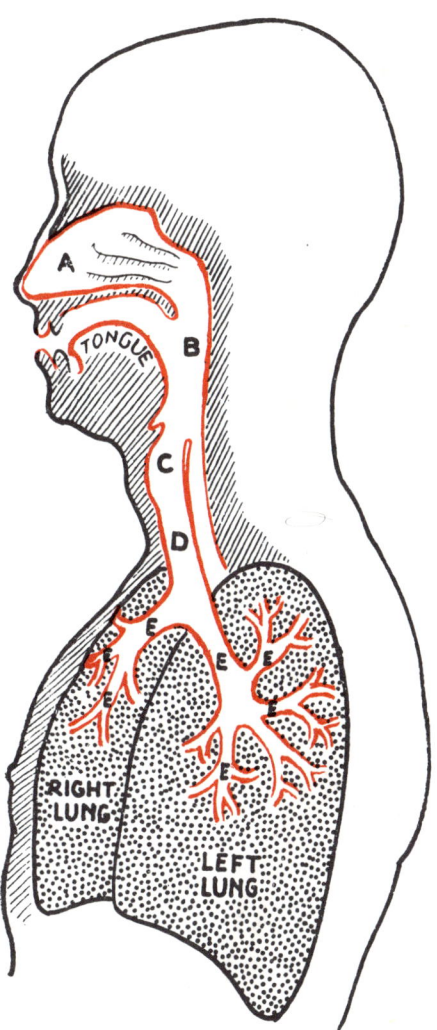

FIGURE 105—Diagram of the air passages
- A—Nasal passage
- B—Pharynx
- C—Larynx
- D—Windpipe
- E—Large and small bronchial tubes

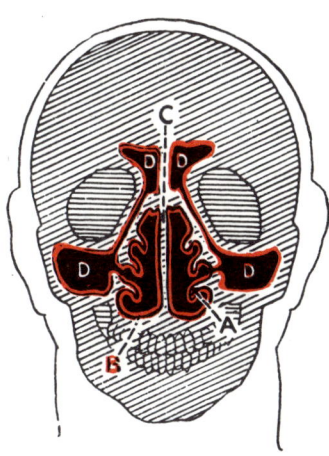

FIGURE 106—A section through the nasal passages diagrammatic)
- A—Bony flange
- B—Mucous membrane
- C—Dividing septum
- D—Sinus

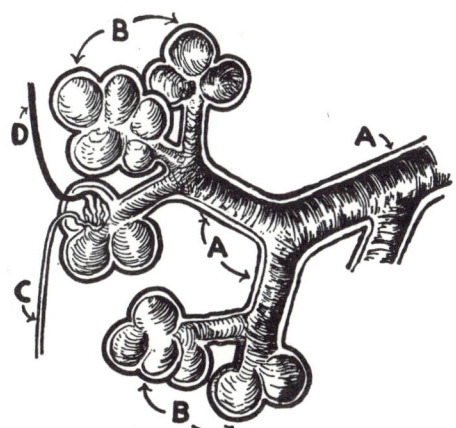

FIGURE 107—Diagram of small bronchial tubes opening into air sacs
- A—Small bronchial tube
- B—Air sac
- C—Arterial end of capillary vessel
- D—Venous end of capillary vessel

The Lungs

The right and left lungs with the heart and large blood vessels occupy most of the thoracic cavity. The substance of the lung is of a light, porous spongy texture and is highly elastic; it consists of millions of air sacs, each opening from a small bronchial tube and having an artery and vein. The walls of an air sac are elastic and are lined by a thin layer of cells; this thin layer separates the blood capillaries in the wall of the sac from the air within the sac and it allows the passage of oxygen from the air sac into the blood capillaries and of carbon dioxide in the reverse direction.

Each lung is covered by a smooth membrane called the *pleura* (Figure 108) which also lines the inner walls of the thorax and the upper aspect of the diaphragm in such a way that it completely encloses the lung, except that part through which the bronchial tubes and blood vessels enter.

The *pleural cavity* is the potential space between the outer and inner layers of the pleura; in normal health this cavity does not exist, because the lungs are in close contact with the chest wall; but if the outer or inner layer of pleura

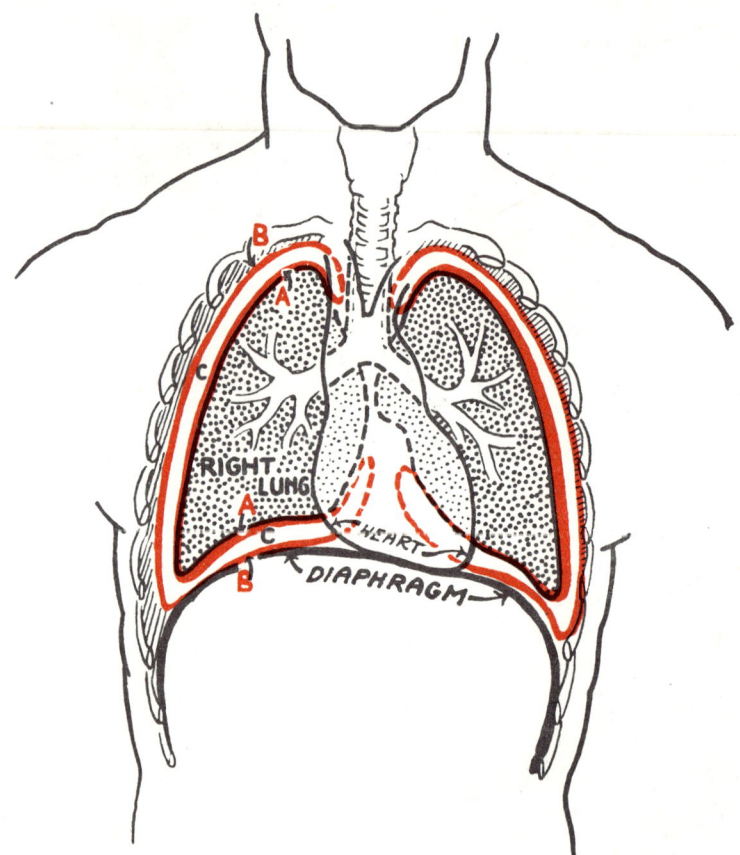

FIGURE 108—Diagram of lungs showing the two layers of pleura (normally the two layers are in contact)
   A—Pleura covering lung
   B—Pleura lining inner wall of thorax
   C—Pleural cavity

is punctured air enters the potential space between the layers and it becomes an actual space as the lung contracts on account of the elastic tissue which it contains. The lung cannot be expanded again until a negative pressure* has been restored, because the thoracic walls and diaphragm have no means of sucking out the surfaces of the lung to draw in air. Fortunately, if one lung has collapsed as a result of the entry of air into its pleural cavity, the other lung is capable of carrying out the function of respiration, because the two pleural cavities are not connected to one another.

Vital Capacity

The vital capacity of an individual can be determined by measuring the maximum amount of air that can be expired after a maximum inspiration. In quiet respiration the lungs are working at about one-tenth of their full capacity, the volume of air passing in and out of the lungs with each breath being between 300 and 500 ccs. (cubic centimetres). This is called the *tidal air*. If after taking a normal breath a maximal inspiratory effort is made the additional air inspired, called the *complemental air*, amounts to about 1,500 ccs. Likewise additional air can be expired from the lungs by a maximal effort after a normal expiration; it is called the *supplemental air* and again amounts to about 1,500 ccs. The sum of the volumes of tidal, complemental and supplemental air is thus the vital capacity, which averages 3,500 ccs. in normal health. It is decreased in certain heart and lung diseases; it may be increased by suitable breathing exercises and athletics.

There is still some air left in the air sacs of the lungs after a maximal expiration; this is called the *residual air*, and its volume is about 1,200 ccs. The air in the air passages, about 150 ccs., is called *dead space air*.

The vital capacity of the lungs is a measure of their ability to respond to the additional oxygen requirements of the body during moderate or severe exercise. A high vital capacity does not necessarily create a greater feeling of fitness, but it permits an active existence. On the other hand a subnormal vital capacity in young people is very often a sign of disease of the heart or lungs.

The Chemistry of Respiration

The air which we breathe into our lungs consists of:
    Oxygen 20.96 per cent.   Nitrogen 79.00 per cent.
                Carbon dioxide 0.04 per cent.

Nitrogen plays no part in respiration other than diluting the oxygen. The relative proportions of these gases remain fairly constant at all altitudes but the higher one goes above sea level the less becomes the density of the air. At 10,000 feet, the atmosphere has only about three-quarters of its sea level density so that the amount of oxygen it contains per cubic foot is correspondingly reduced. Under such conditions the body at rest can obtain sufficient oxygen by increasing the rate of respiration, but at heights above 15,000 feet, oxygen is not present in sufficient quantity to satisfy body needs even though the rate of respiration is further increased. At 30,000 feet there is so little oxygen that a person in an aircraft not wearing an oxygen mask would become unconscious in a very short time.

The effect of a mild degree of oxygen lack is rather similar to that produced by an over indulgence in alcohol. Judgment and understanding are much impaired and body sensations dulled; but the subject is not himself aware of these changes and is convinced that his mind is clear and that he is capable of dealing with any situation. Such a state of mind in persons flying in aircraft is obviously a source of great danger. So much emphasis has been laid upon the importance of oxygen when flying over 10,000 feet that all members of air crews have now become completely oxygen minded.

* Negative pressure is a term which means pressure less than that exerted by the atmosphere, which is 15 pounds to the square inch. This atmospheric pressure is exerted all over the body surface and of course inside the lungs as well, because the air passages are in direct communication with the outside air.

The air which we breathe out of our lungs contains about 16 per cent. oxygen and 4 per cent. carbon dioxide. The mechanism of the gaseous exchange in the lungs is too complicated to explain in detail, but some idea of the principle involved may be obtained by considering the action of a soda syphon. In a syphon, water and a gas (carbon dioxide) are mixed under pressure; some of the gas dissolves in the water until an equilibrium has been reached between the gas in the water and the gas above it. If some soda water is withdrawn, upward streams of bubbles immediately appear in great quantities in the water in the syphon. The reason for this is that the pressure of the gas above the water has been reduced, so upsetting the equilibrium; the dissolved gas therefore starts to leave the water and continues to do so until an equilibrium is once more established. The same thing occurs in the soda water which has been withdrawn; the carbon dioxide rapidly bubbles out of the water until the pressure of the gas in the water is the same as that in the air*.

The gases dissolved in the blood, oxygen and carbon dioxide, behave in a similar way. When venous blood reaches the lungs, it contains a lower percentage of oxygen and a higher percentage of carbon dioxide than contained by the air in the lungs. Oxygen therefore diffuses through the walls of the air sacs and is taken up by the haemoglobin in the blood; carbon dioxide passes from the blood into the air sacs whence it is removed by normal respiration.

Expired air contains a considerable amount of water vapour in addition to carbon dioxide; this water vapour can be seen on a cold day as small clouds condensing from the breath. Much heat is lost in the water vapour.

SECTION 3—THE ALIMENTARY TRACT

The alimentary tract is a tubular structure which begins at the mouth and ends at the anus. It guides and controls the passage of food through the body and has mechanisms for ingestion, digestion, absorption and ultimate excretion.

The Mouth (Figure 109)

The tongue, teeth and salivary glands prepare the food before it reaches the stomach. The saliva is secreted into the sides and floor of the mouth through ducts; it has a slight digestive action, but its main function is to act as a lubricant to make easy the chewing and swallowing of food. The thought, sight or appetizing smell of food starts the secretion of saliva.

The Gullet

This is a narrow muscular tube about ten inches long connecting the pharynx to the stomach. It passes behind the windpipe and the heart and through the diaphragm into the stomach. The walls at its upper end are composed of voluntary muscle and at its lower end of involuntary muscle. The entry of food into the lungs is prevented by the *epiglottis* which is closed automatically over the entrance into the larynx, like a trap-door, whenever food is swallowed.

The Stomach

The stomach is the widest part of the alimentary tract; it is a muscular organ situated in the upper half of the abdomen mostly on the left side. immediately below the diaphragm and heart. It varies greatly in position and shape according to the amount it contains and the position of the body. Its walls are composed of three criss-crossing layers of involuntary muscle fibres and it has a thick lining of mucous membrane containing the glands which secrete the gastric juice.

The narrow, lower end of the stomach, called the *pylorus*, is thickened by a circular layer of involuntary muscle which by contraction can close the exit from the stomach. The pylorus is usually closed, but during digestion it opens periodically to allow the onward passage of food into the intestine.

* As already mentioned the percentage of carbon dioxide in the air is very small: for this reason bottled beer may be prevented from going flat if the stopper is firmly screwed in, thus maintaining the concentration of carbon dioxide.

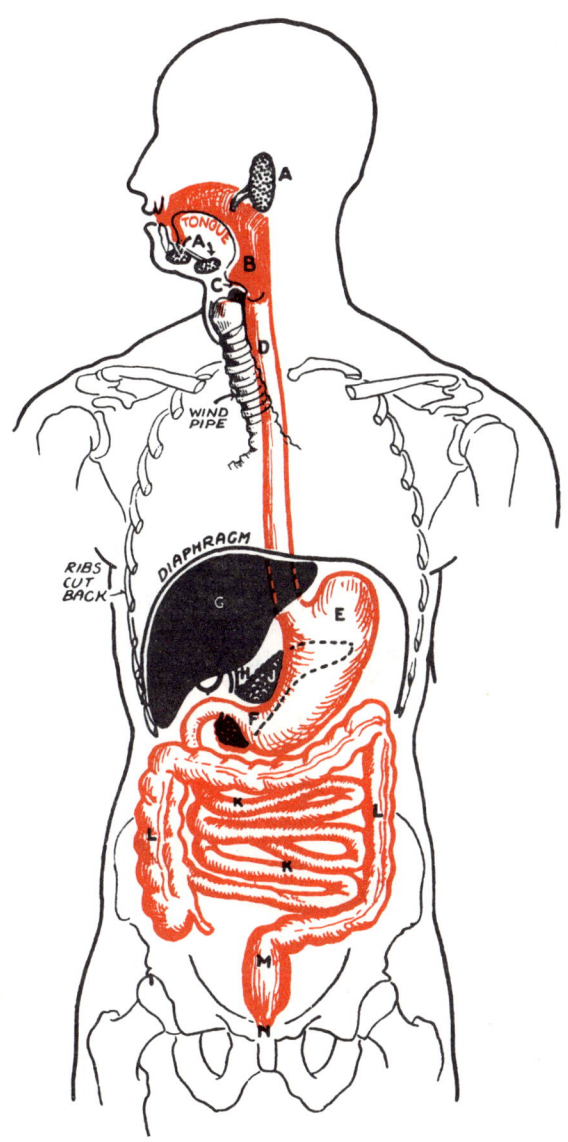

FIGURE 109—The alimentary tract (diagrammatic)

A—Salivary glands E—Upper end of stomach J—Pancreas
B—Pharynx F—Pylorus K—Small intestine
C—Epiglottis G—Liver L—Large intestine
D—Gullet H—Bile duct M—Rectum
　　　　　　　　N—Anal canal

The Intestine

The intestine is divided into two parts of differing diameter; the first part is called the *small intestine* and the second part the *large intestine*.

The *small intestine* is about 22 feet long and one inch in diameter. It has two layers of involuntary muscle in its walls and is lined by a layer of mucous membrane containing numerous glands which secrete digestive juices. The mucous membrane is thrown into many folds to increase the surface area for absorption.

The upper end of the small intestine is joined by a duct formed by the junction of two other ducts, one from the liver, the bile duct, which conveys bile from the gall bladder to the small intestine, and the other from the pancreas, a glandular organ which secretes digestive juices (see paragraph on digestion).

The *large intestine* is about 4 feet long and has an average diameter of two inches. It begins in the lower right side of the abdominal cavity and passes up the right side, across the upper part and down the left side into the pelvis where it widens out to form the *rectum*; the narrow passage leading from the rectum is called the *anal canal*. The structure of the walls of the large intestine is similar to that of the small intestine, but its mucous membrane contains mucous glands only, which secrete a lubricating fluid. The stomach and intestines are supported in the abdominal cavity by a double layer of membrane called the *mesentery* (Figure 110); it is part of the membrane which lines the whole abdominal cavity.

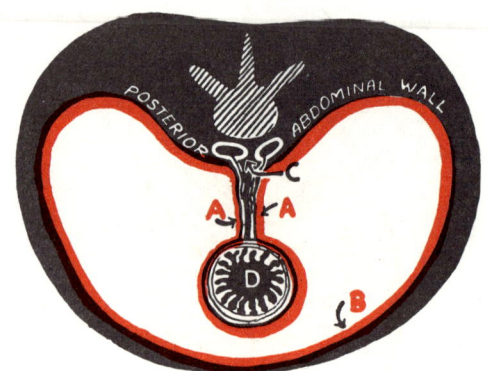

FIGURE 110—Section through abdominal cavity showing method of suspension of the gut to the posterior abdominal wall (diagrammatic)

A—Mesentery   C—Vessels
B—Membrane lining abdomen   D—Gut

The mesentery keeps the stomach and intestines anchored to the posterior abdominal wall. The blood vessels, of which there are a very great number, pass to and from the gut between the two layers of the mesentery.

Food

A diet which contains all the foodstuffs necessary to maintain the body in health would be made up of the following components:

(1) *proteins*;
(2) *carbohydrates*;
(3) *fats*;
(4) *water*;
(5) *vitamins*;
(6) *minerals*.

(1) *Proteins* are chemical compounds made up mainly of *nitrogen, carbon, hydrogen* and *oxygen* in varying proportions. Meat, cheese, fish, peas and beans are very rich in proteins; milk, bread, butter and eggs contain rather less and vegetables and fruits very little. The muscles, skin, internal organs and other soft tissues are composed mainly of protein substances.

(2) *Carbohydrates* are made up of varying proportions of carbon, hydrogen and oxygen. Sugar is a pure carbohydrate; bread, cereals, potatoes and other root vegetables contain a large amount. Carbohydrates are substances which are readily convertible into energy.

(3) *Fats* are chiefly derived from animal sources; examples are butter, cheese, eggs and animal fat itself. Fat performs several functions in the diet:
    (i) it can act as a source of energy;
    (ii) it can be readily stored to act as an energy reserve;
    (iii) it provides certain vitamins essential for health and growth.

(4) *Water* is contained in varying proportions in most carbohydrate and protein foodstuffs. Vegetable foodstuffs contain a very high percentage of water. Protein foodstuffs such as meat contain somewhat less. If for example a pound of lean meat is chemically analysed about two-thirds of a pound of water can be extracted.

(5) *Vitamins* are complex substances which are essential for life, health and growth. They assist in various ways the many chemical reactions which occur in the body, but they are not themselves a source of energy. The chief known vitamins are A, B, C and D.

Vitamin A is found in fats of animal origin, that is, in milk, cream, butter, liver, eggs and in very large concentrations in cod and halibut liver oil. It is found in vegetables such as carrots, spinach and tomatoes. A severe deficiency of vitamin A may have many ill effects on the general health: the resistance to infection is greatly reduced and there is an increased susceptibility to respiratory infections and inflammation of the eyes; night blindness and diminished acuity of vision may also occur. The skin becomes dry and shrivelled and is liable to develop infections. The normal diet usually contains an adequate quantity of vitamin A and is it only in exceptional circumstances that the conditions mentioned above occur.

Vitamin B is found in most seeds, for example, wheat, pulses, yeast, peanuts barley and rice and in eggs. A prolonged deficiency of this vitamin causes intestinal disturbances, and also certain forms of nerve and skin troubles (beri-beri, pellagra).

Vitamin C is found in fresh fruits and vegetables such as blackcurrants, oranges, lemons, apples, tomatoes, lettuce and raw cabbage leaves. Milk contains a small quantity. If this vitamin is absent from the diet for long, *scurvy* develops; in this condition there is bleeding beneath the skin and from the gums, the walls of the intestine and the kidneys. Sailors frequently suffered from this disease years ago when voyages occupied many months and fresh fruit was not available, until they learnt that this disease was preventable if fruits such as lemons and oranges were added to the diet.* A deficiency is occasionally seen in babies which have been fed on artificial food exclusively for six or seven months.

Vitamin D is found in fish liver oil and in eggs. It is essential for the normal growth of bone and without it *rickets* develop, in which the bones become soft owing to a lack of lime salts and the process of growth, which takes place at the ends of the bones, is disturbed. Administration of adequate doses of vitamin D cures the condition.

The ultra-violet rays in sunlight may be used in the treatment of rickets. When they are directed on to the bare skin, they convert a certain inactive

---

* In Treasure Island it is recorded that a barrel of apples was kept on deck to prevent scurvy. The choice of this fruit was unfortunate for it contains least vitamin C of all the commoner fruits and vegetables.

substance in it into an active substance which has all the properties of the vitamin.

Nowadays we are constantly told by advertisements that vitamins are necessary for our health. This true statement misleads many people, as the advertisers intend. In fact the diet consumed by the average person contains enough of the necessary vitamins, but many people, believing they are doing without something essential to them, consume large quantities of patent foods and medicines. A good all round mixed diet, with plenty of fresh fruit or vegetables, contains all the vitamins we need. Vitamin concentrates should not be added to it without medical advice.

(6) The minerals needed by the body are chiefly *common salt, calcium, phosphorus, iron* and *iodine*. A deficiency of any of these substances leads to a general disturbance of normal function. Calcium and phosphorus are present in fairly large quantities in milk; iron is obtained from meat, vegetables and fruits. Traces of iodine are present in drinking water in almost all parts of the United Kingdom.

Digestion

The preliminary stages of the digestion of food begin in the mouth, where saliva has a slight action on cooked starches, such as potato. Thorough mastication of food is important because the digestive juices can then act upon it more easily, making both digestion and absorption more efficient. When the food has been thoroughly masticated the tongue shapes it against the roof of the mouth into a pellet called a *bolus*; the bolus is swallowed and passes down the gullet into the stomach. On reaching the stomach it is thoroughly mixed with the acid gastric juices and the digestion of proteins is begun; the gastric juices destroy most of the bacteria which contaminate the food.

The stomach begins to discharge its contents into the small intestine about half an hour after the food is swallowed and is normally quite empty after about three hours. When the acid contents from the stomach enter the small intestine, they are neutralised by the alkaline juices secreted by the glands of the intestine; further secretions, namely bile and pancreatic juices, are poured into the upper end of the small intestine as the food passes through. The bile contains special salts which help digestion of fats; the pancreas provides three different secretions which help digestion of proteins, fats and carbohydrates.

The food takes about two hours to pass through the small intestine, and during that time insoluble substances are converted into soluble ones which can be absorbed through the walls of the intestine and carried away by the circulation to nourish the body.

By the time the contents reach the large intestine digestion is complete. Up to the time of entering into the large intestine the food residue is quite fluid, but during its passage through the large intestine most of the remaining water is absorbed. When the contents of the large bowel reach the rectum, they remain there until expelled by the act of defaecation. The total time which elapses in health between the ingestion of food and its arrival in the rectum is never much less than eighteen hours.

Movement of food through the alimentary tract is started by the voluntary act of swallowing. As soon as the food reaches the lower part of the gullet its movement comes under the control of involuntary muscle fibres which contract behind it and squeeze it onward towards the stomach. In the same way food passes through the stomach and intestine under the control of involuntary muscle until it reaches the rectum.

The blood collects in the numerous vessels supplying the stomach and intestines during digestion; if it is diverted away from these parts digestion will cease or be inefficiently carried out. When vigorous activity is taken immediately after a meal, the blood is diverted away from the gut by a nervous mechanism to increase the supply to the muscles; the digestive process is thus interrupted. At least one hour should be allowed to elapse after a meal before starting any vigorous exercise. Anger or excitement during a meal will also have an adverse effect on digestion for the same reason.

Energy Requirements

The energy value of foods is measured in heat units called Calories.* The reason for using this type of measuremnt may be explained by the following example. If a piece of metal is filed, both the metal and the file become hot; the mechanical energy provided by the muscles performing the work is converted into heat energy; the muscle energy has not disappeared but has reappeared in the form of heat; energy is indestructible and one form can therefore be measured in terms of another. The energy values of different kinds of food have been determined by burning the food in a special apparatus called a calorimeter, the amount of heat liberated being expressed in Calories.

A diet must have a Calorie value large enough to provide the energy requirements of the body. A man doing light manual work or sedentary work, which includes all kinds of brain work, requires about 3,000 Calories every twenty-four hours; a woman requires about 10 per cent. less. These requirements depend, in the adult, on the surface area of the body and the type of work performed; children require relatively more than an adult. Persons performing very heavy manual work need as much as 5,000 Calories every twenty-four hours. One possible way of supplying a man's Calorie requirements is shown in the following specimen diet for twenty-four hours. There are of course many others.

		Calorie value
Porridge	2 oz. dry	212
Bacon	2 oz.	250
Eggs	2 oz.	45
Sugar	½ oz.	56
Marmalade	½ oz.	45
Butter	½ oz.	106
Bread (white)	12 oz.	900
Beef, mutton	3 oz.	200
Boiled potatoes	10 oz.	210
Greens	8 oz.	56
Orange, apple	3 oz.	36
Cod	4 oz.	75
Cheese	1 oz.	112
Biscuits	1 oz.	117
Milk†	1 pint	340
Jam	½ oz.	30
Fats in cooking	½ oz.	100
Beer	1 pint	200
	Total	3090 Calories

All rationing schemes should be based on physiological requirements. At the end of the first world war an attempt was made by some mid-European countries to maintain the people's daily diet at a value of 2,500 Calories, with slightly more for heavy workers. No ill effects were noticed for some time, but after several months there was a marked falling off in the general health of the people and an increased susceptibility to disease. As a result of the second world war the diet of certain European countries was for long periods deficient in essential foodstuffs, particularly fats and proteins, a deficiency in the latter causing muscle weakness. As would be expected the incidence of tuberculosis and other respiratory infections was extremely high in these countries.

* A calorie is the amount of heat required to raise the temperature of 1 ml. of water 1 degree Centigrade. The Calorie to which reference is made above is the large Calorie and is 1,000 times greater than the small calorie.

† Tea without milk or sugar has no calorie value.

SECTION 4—THE EXCRETORY SYSTEM

The waste products of tissue activity are excreted through the body by one or other of the following organs:
  (1) the anal canal;
  (2) the kidneys;
  (3) the skin;
  (4) the lungs.

The excretion of carbon dioxide and water from the lungs has already been described; in health no other substance except alcohol is excreted through the lungs. In disease the body may rid itself of many pathological products through the lungs; apart from disease, certain drugs, particularly volatile anæsthetics, such as ether, or narcotics, such as paraldehyde, are normally excreted mainly or partly through the lungs.

The excretion of undigestible food residue through the anal canal has also been described; bile pigment formed in the liver from the haemoglobin of worn out red cells is excreted in the faeces and gives them their characteristic colour. Many other substances too varied to enumerate and too intricate in their biological chemistry to describe are also excreted through the anal canal. Of the other two organs mentioned above the kidneys are by far the more important.

The two kidneys lie one each side of the vertebral column on the posterior wall of the abdominal cavity. Each kidney consists of two layers of tissue, an outer and an inner, called the *cortex* and *medulla* respectively. It is supplied by an artery and a vein, and a tube, called the *ureter*, connects it with the urinary bladder. Its tissue is built up of thousands of excretory units, called *glomeruli*, each supplied by a small artery and vein and connected with the ureter by a long tube which has many loops. The glomerulus consists essentially of a tuft of blood vessels covered by a capsule lined by special cells which have a selective action and allow only certain substances in the blood, such as sugar and salt, to filter through into the tubular portion. The glomeruli and part of their tubular attachments are situated in the cortex; the rest of the tubular apparatus is in the medulla.

The watery fluid filtered by the glomeruli contains common salt, urea and uric acid; it does not contain any protein or fat. In its passage down the tubes, water and common salt are absorbed in quantities in accord with the need of the body. On a hot day a man who has taken vigorous exercise, without fluid refreshment, passes a highly coloured and concentrated urine in which the salt content is low. Both water and salt are required by the skin for sweating. On the other hand when, on a cold day, he has had several pints of beer, he passes large quantities of dilute urine to excrete the water which his body does not need.

The kidney also excretes many other substances and makes use of complicated methods in so doing. These matters are not of present interest, but it is important not to assume that the very brief and bald account given above, though true, does justice to the delicate and fascinating mechanism of excretion by the kidney of which only a little is yet known.

The salt and water are excreted as sweat through the skin. The openings of the sweat glands can be seen with a magnifying glass on the surface of the skin; they look like small pits and are found in greatest concentration on the hairless parts, such as the forehead and the palms of the hands. Sweat is excreted rapidly in hot weather or after strenuous exercise and may be seen as drops on the skin; as it evaporates the skin is cooled*. Sweating is associated with an

---

* A fixed amount of energy in the form of heat is required to convert a given quantity of a liquid into vapour. The vaporization of sweat removes energy in the form of heat from the skin and in so doing cools it.

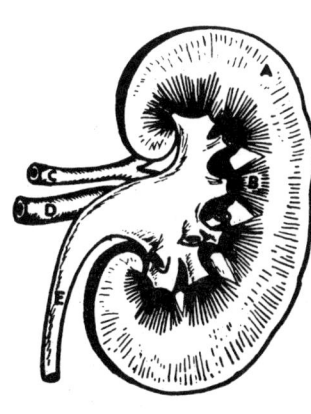
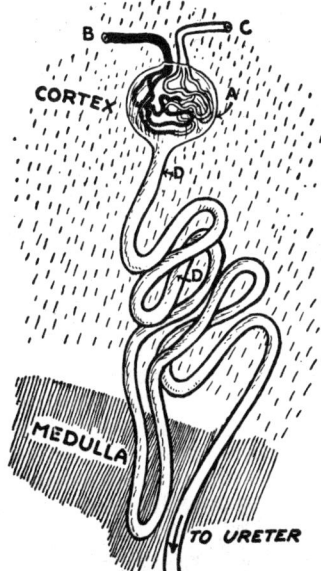

FIGURE 111—Section through kidney
A—Cortex   C—Artery
B—Medulla D—Vein
E—Ureter

FIGURE 112—Diagram of glomerulus and tube (greatly enlarged)
A—Glomerulus   C—Vein
B—Artery   D—Tubule

increased output of carbon dioxide by the skin, which may therefore be regarded as an unimportant but alternative route for the excretion of that substance.

The real importance of sweating lies in its influence on the temperature of the body, which normally loses heat in three ways, *radiation, conduction* and *evaporation*. If the temperature of the surrounding air is the same as that of the body, heat can then only be lost by the evaporation of sweat. The dry heat of a Turkish bath can cause the loss of over 5 pounds of body weight in two and a half hours, almost all being lost in sweat.

Stokers and miners frequently suffer from painful contractions in their muscles; this is a sign that they have been losing too much salt from their bodies as a result of continuous and profuse sweating in a warm, dry atmosphere The condition is known as *heat cramp* and can be prevented by taking additional salt-containing fluids in the diet.

SECTION 5— THE NERVOUS SYSTEM

The nervous system is the highly complex mechanism by which man reacts to his environment and co-ordinates his mental and bodily activities. It consists of the *brain*, protected by the skull, the *spinal cord*, protected by the vertebrae which form a special canal for it, and the *peripheral*, free running nerves which supply all parts of the body. In addition, there are small masses of nervous tissue in various parts of the body, usually near the brain or spinal cord.

The brain is the centre of appreciation, where all incoming messages, whether entering consciousness or not, are analysed and appropriate action is initiated; the spinal chord groups, transmits and relays messages to and from the brain, and the peripheral nerves transmit messages between the spinal cord and the general body tissues.

The nervous system may be compared with a complicated telephone network, and the brain with the central exchange itself. Messages are sent from all parts of the body about pressure, pain, temperature, touch and position, and from the ears, eyes, nose and mouth; they are rapidly sorted, interpreted and correlated in the brain which then relays information and instruction throughout the body.

The brain and spinal cord together are called, for convenience, the *central nervous system*. The free nerves, running from the central nervous system to all other parts of the body, make up the *peripheral nervous system*; this classification is an anatomical one.

Structure of Nervous Tissue

Nervous tissue consists essentially of nerve cells and their branches, supported by connective tissues. Nerve cells (Figure 114) differ widely in shape and size; they have a nucleus, several small branches called *dendrites* for the reception of messages, and normally one branch, the *axon* or nerve fibre for their transmission. A nerve cell with its branches forms the basic unit of the nervous system and is called a *neurone*. Most axons, or nerve fibres, are covered by two sheaths; the outer is a thin membrane and the inner is made up of a white fatty substance. The inner membrane appears white and glistening and the masses of nerve fibres covered with it constitute the *white matter* of the nervous system. The cell body and its dendrites have no membrane and are grey. The popular phrase 'grey matter' has thus a sound anatomical basis, because the grey part of the nervous system contains the bodies of the cells where thought processes occur, but the white parts contain only the nerve fibres or mere telephone wires. The peripheral nerves are made up almost entirely of axons, and are therefore white.

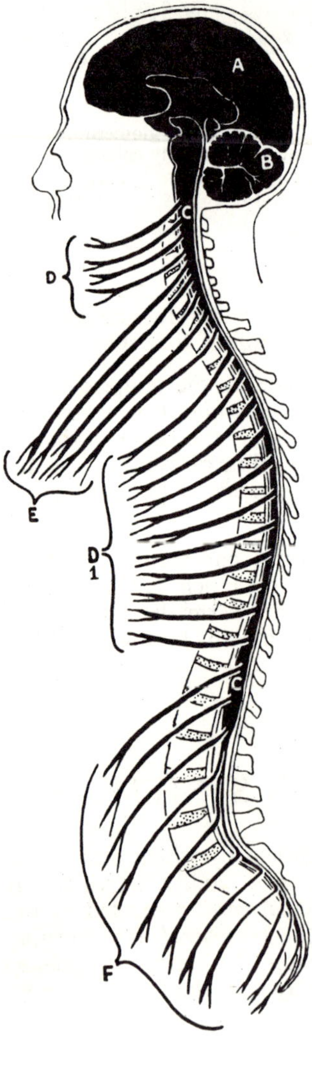

FIGURE 113—The central and peripheral nervous systems (diagrammatic)

A—Cerebrum
B—Cerebellum } forming central nervous system
D—Spinal cord
D—Peripheral nerves supplying structures on the left side of the neck
D¹—Peripheral nerves supplying structures of left side of thorax and abdomen
E and F—Peripheral nerves to upper and lower limbs respectively

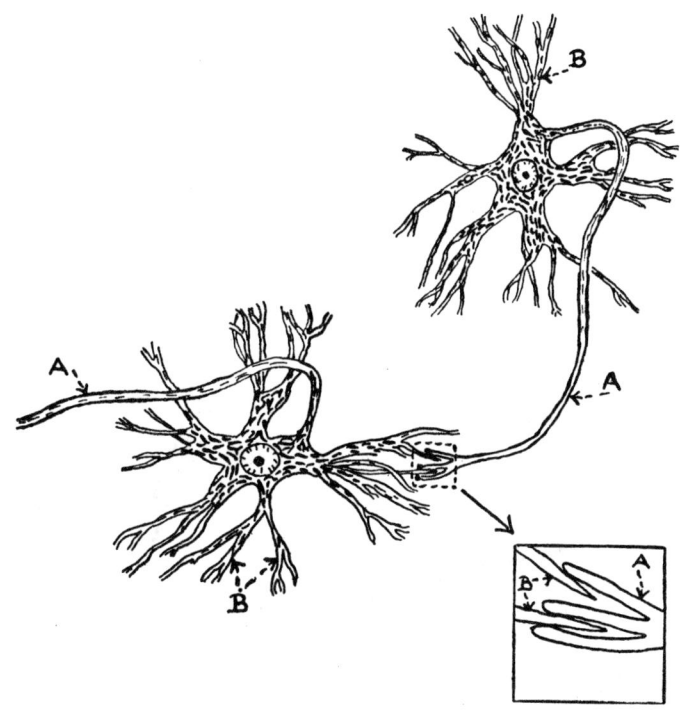

FIGURE 114—Two nerve cells
A—Axons
B—Dendrites

Inset—A *diagram* of the meeting between axon and dendrites, showing the contact but anatomical separateness which is called a *synapse*

Function of Nervous Tissue

The characteristic function of nervous tissue is the carrying of nervous impulses. Nervous tissue reacts to almost any stimulus as a result of its highly developed excitability. The exact nature of a nervous impulse is not known, but it has many characteristics identical with those of a simple electric current. Electricity is commonly used to excite nervous impulses under experimental conditions, but the electricity itself is not conducted through the nerve fibres; the rate of conduction of a nervous impulse in man is between 30 and 90 metres per second, according to the type of nerve fibre. This rate is many hundreds of thousands of times less than the rate of conduction of electricity.

The Structure of a Free Nerve

Nerve fibres retain their two sheaths when they leave the central nervous system, and they are bound together into bundles: a great number of these bundles together form a free or *peripheral* nerve. Such a nerve may be felt at the elbow joint as it passes round the inner portion of the lower end of the humerus; this is the *ulnar* nerve. Some of the effects of pressure on a nerve can be demonstrated by rolling the ulnar nerve hard against the bone. 'Pins and needles' are felt in the ring and little fingers. Such sensations are more keenly felt when the ulnar nerve is accidently compressed against the upper and inner part of the ulna. This is popularly known as knocking the 'funny bone'.

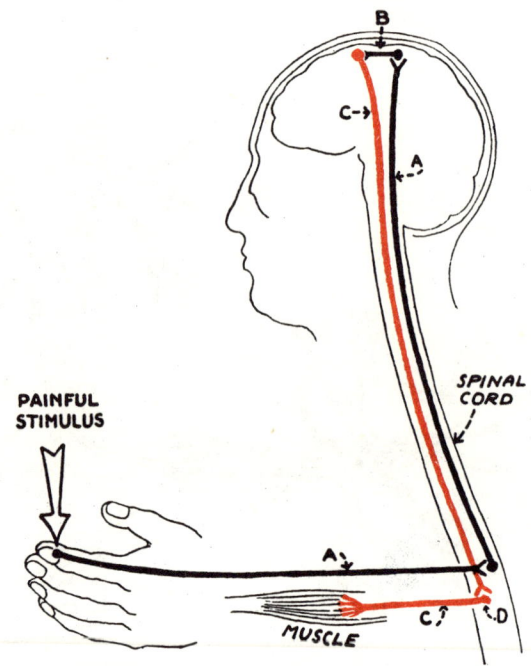

FIGURE 115—Simplified diagram showing path of sensory and motor neurones
    A—Sensory neurone (afferent)
    B—Intercommunicating branch between cells in grey matter
    C—Motor neurone to muscle (efferent)
    D—Anterior horn cell in grey matter of spinal cord

The nerves which carry impulses away from the brain are called *efferent* nerves, and those which convey sensations to it are called *afferent* nerves. They are similar except for their endings. Most of the efferent nerves are *motor nerves* and most of the *afferent* nerves are *sensory nerves* (Figure 115).

A *motor* nerve ends in the muscle it supplies and transmits impulses to the muscle fibres, causing them to contract. A *sensory* nerve has highly sensitive endings in the skin, muscles or joints; sensory impulses are conveyed through it to the brain, where the sensation is appreciated, although the sensation is felt at the site from which the impulses are brought. An area of skin becomes anaesthetic or devoid of feeling if the sensory nerve connecting it to the brain is cut.

The nerves which supply involuntary muscle as, for example, those in the walls of the intestines or the blood vessels, are constructed in a similar fashion and for the most part their fibres run with the fibres of the sensory and motor nerves.

Function of the Nervous System

Functionally the nervous system may be considered under three headings.*
    (1) The involuntary system.
    (2) The sensorimotor system.
    (3) The reflex and intercommunicating system.

The *involuntary system* is the basic nervous system upon which later refinements of nervous structure and action were built. It is represented in man by the *sympathetic* nervous system and the *parasympathetic* nervous system. These two systems are mutually antagonistic.

The sympathetic nervous system is a general activator of all the tissues in the body whose functions are vital for a satisfactory response to excitement

* Naturally in the body there are no such artificial divisions; the classification is merely one of convenience.

or danger. Its activities can best be shown be describing what happens when a man gets a bad fright. The fear is appreciated intellectually and emotionally by the brain, which sets the machinery of the sympathetic system in motion. Partly by nervous stimulation and partly by chemical action produced by nervous stimulation, the heart beats more quickly and strongly, blood is removed from the skin and the bowel and shunted to the brain and muscles, digestion ceases, and the breathing becomes deeper. Smaller signs of this state are the hair standing on end and the dilatation of the pupil; as the ghost in Hamlet aptly says, fright makes 'each particular hair to stand on end, like quills upon the fretful porcupine.'

The parasympathetic system, on the other hand, permits a vegetative state rather like sitting and thinking or just sitting—the perfect picture of man after a full dinner. The parasympathetic nerves reduce the volume and output of the heart, check the rate and depth of respiration, shunt blood passively to the bowel and encourage the process of digestion and the secretion of digestive juices.

The sympathetic and parasympathetic systems between them are also responsible for the automatic control of other more complex mechanisms; for example, *micturition*, or passing water, *defaecation*, or passing faeces, and *parturition*, or giving birth.

The *sensorimotor system* subserves sensation and movement. Two large areas on each side of the brain are concerned entirely with the appreciation of sensation and the initiation of movement. These areas are situated in the forebrain, or *cerebrum*, which was the latest part of the nervous system to develop. Thought and all other mental activities connected with sensation and movement are also carried out in the cerebrum. Two large bundles of nerve fibres from each side of the cerebrum traverse the lower part of the brain and brain stem and pass into the spinal cord, each individual fibre ending at a nerve cell somewhere in the cord. The cells at which these fibres from the brain end, give rise to axons which pass in bundles through the intervertebral spaces to form the peripheral nerves (Figure 113).

There are thirty-one pairs of nerves which arise from the spine in this way and twelve others, called *cranial* nerves, which arise from the brain stem in much the same way, to supply various structures in the head and neck.

The nerve fibres which carry motor impulses from the brain end in the anterior part of the spinal cord; the cells which relay the messages further via the peripheral nerves are situated in the anterior grey matter of the spinal cord.

Sensory impulses from the skin and other structures pass up the peripheral nerves to the cells in the posterior grey matter, whence they are relayed up the posterior part of the spinal cord to the sensory area of the brain.

The fibres from the cells of the anterior grey matter and the posterior grey matter of the cord leave in two separate bundles, which join outside the cord to form the peripheral nerves, which are therefore known as mixed motor and sensory nerves. These mixed nerves are joined by fibres from the involuntary system, whose nerve centres are those mentioned in the introduction to this section as lying near the spinal cord.

It must be emphasised that the *reflex and intercommunicating nervous system* is not a separate and discrete mass of nervous tissue, but is inextricably mixed with the sensorimotor and involuntary systems; its separation here is purely to make easy the explanation of its function.

However, there are parts of the central nervous system almost exclusively serving reflex action.

Reflex action is a reaction to a sensory impulse; it is brought about through the medium of the central nervous system, where the sensory impulse produces a motor response, with or without obtrusion upon consciousness.

A simple and important reflex action occurs when the tendon of the quadriceps is quickly stretched by a smart tap; the proper way to elicit this reflex is to cross one leg over the other, stretching the quadriceps and its tendon in so doing, and then to tap the tendon just below the patella. The nervous impulses pass through a circuit called the *reflex arc* in the manner described below.

The tap stretches the tendon and the muscle, both of which have specialised nerve endings which are sensitive to stretching. Impulses pass up through the afferent nerve fibres from these nerve endings to the spinal cord. Here the information that the tendon and muscle have been stretched is relayed from the posterior grey matter to the anterior grey matter in the cells of which a new nervous impulse arises; this impulse passes through efferent fibres to the quadriceps muscle, which contracts as a result. At the same time messages are sent within the spinal cord to the anterior grey matter, which controls the activity of the hamstring muscles which, it will be remembered, act in opposition to the quadriceps. The effect of these messages is to make the hamstring muscles relax during the contraction of the quadriceps.

This reflex, the knee jerk, is a very simple one and utilises only afferent and efferent peripheral nerves, and the spinal cord in the lumbar and sacral regions. Other reflex actions, though apparently simple, may be very complicated and require the help of nervous tissue in the brain stem and in the part of the brain behind the brain stem and cerebrum called the *cerebellum* or little brain. The cerebellum is almost entirely concerned with reflex action at a high functional level.

The Nervous Control of Posture

Waiting in a queue may seem a simple if tedious procedure, but it can be made to illustrate many of the nervous and muscular actions performed and controlled automatically by the reflex and intercommunicating nervous system.

At first, a woman standing in a queue knows that she is standing there, but soon she begins to think of other things. The pressure of the pavement transmitted to the soles of her feet ceases to impress itself upon consciousness but she does not therefore fall down; on the contrary, she remains standing where she was.

The nervous impulses from the soles of the feet do not all travel up the sensory pathway to the cerebrum; many of them are sent to centres in the spinal cord, the brain stem and the cerebellum. Those which travel no higher than the cord give information which is used by the cells of the anterior grey matter to relax or contract groups of muscles such as the muscles of the calf, which plantar flex the ankle to tilt the body backward when they contract. Those which travel to the brain stem are received by centres which are also informed by other nervous impulses from the eyes, the balancing organs behind the ears, and the muscles and tendons of the trunk and neck, of the positions of the head and trunk in relation to the external world. The centres in the brain stem take some action themselves by passing instructions down to the anterior grey matter of the spinal cord which guides and assists the muscle group of the legs by a further series of nervous impulses. Much of the information from the brain stem however, passes to the cerebellum, apart from the information which arises from all the structures previously mentioned, the spinal cord, and the soles of the feet themselves.

To sum up: the spinal cord is permitted some freedom of action on the basis of the information which it receives, but it is controlled by the brain stem which is given much fuller information. In turn the brain stem is controlled by the cerebellum which has at its disposal all the available information from every appropriate organ or structure in the body.

The methods used by the nervous system to maintain the upright position of the body without conscious effort are not substantially different from those which it uses to maintain other postures or produce the components of complicated movement. A further example may serve to explain simply how the reflex and intercommunicating nervous system aids the performance of voluntary movements.

A person standing by the light of a window to thread a needle is wholly absorbed in guiding the thread through the narrow eye. The positions of the legs, trunk, head and neck are controlled in the way already described, but the position of the arms in space and the movements of the hands and eyes are under the active voluntary control of the cerebrum. The position of the arms relative to the shoulders, which may be called the posture of the arms, is however controlled by a nervous mechanism which does not obtrude upon consciousness; it would be a nuisance if it did because the attention would then be divided and not wholly concentrated upon the task in hand.

This posture of the arms has already been decided upon by the cerebrum as an appropriate one for the job, and the cerebrum has given, as it were, general instructions to the cerebellum and brain stem and has left the details to them. The arms are therefore set wholly at the shoulder joint and partly at the elbow joint, leaving the wrist and fingers free to move. The cerebellum and brain stem, 'knowing' from previous experience the pattern of the action, are at once made aware by afferent nervous impulses from the joints, muscles and tendons, of any tendency of the arms to waver, and correcting efferent impulses are sent to maintain the existing position.

The nervous Co-ordination of Muscle Action

A muscle which is carrying out a voluntary movement is called an *agonist* or *prime mover*: the muscle which 'opposes' the movement is called an *antagonist*.* Brachialis and biceps brachialis are the agonists when the elbow is flexed, triceps is the antagonist. During the movement triceps is relaxed by special inhibitory impulses to the cells of the anterior grey matter in the chord which supply it; these impulses damp down the pull of the muscle. This is only one example of co-ordination in muscular action—all the muscle groups of the body are controlled in this way according to the movements which are being performed.

Certain movements require a steady base upon which they may be performed. For example, unscrewing a nut with the fingers requires a fixed wrist so that power may be applied through the ends of the fingers. This fixation of the wrist, and incidentally of the arm, shoulder and the rest of the body, is undertaken by various muscle groups; the muscles which move the wrist, including those which flex and extend it, are contracted to hold the joint rigidly in the most favourable position; muscles which perform such an action to help other muscles are called *synergists*. Almost every movement performed by any part of the body requires the action of synergists for its proper operation.

It is clear that balanced muscle contraction is intimately related to posture and co-ordinated movement, and it is also clear that contraction of muscle fibres in a group of agonists must be counteracted by an equal contraction of muscle fibres in the antagonists, if no movement at the appropriate joint is to occur. For example, if the elbow joint is held flexed at right angles, having just so many fibres contracting in the agonists and antagonists as are necessary to maintain the elbow in that condition, then both groups of muscles are balanced; but if the arm is extended, the number of fibres contracting in the extensors is increased, and the number of fibres contracting in the flexors is decreased. This involves the antagonists in a controlled relaxation or paying out the slack mechanism.

The contraction of muscles is one of the main sources of body heat. There is a nervous centre in the brain which is concerned with the regulation of temperature, and it can influence the nervous tissue governing the muscles and produce active muscle contraction when the body is cold. This is the act of shivering.

* The word antagonist rather suggests that it opposes the action of the agonist, but, in fact, it does everything to facilitate the action.

Muscle tone is an inherent property of normally innervated muscles at rest. The precise mechanism of this is not understood, but it does not appear to represent an active contraction of individual muscle fibres in the sense of the previous paragraphs. Muscle tone is abolished by cutting the nerve supply to a muscle and is also absent in some neurological conditions.

The Cranial Nerves

The twelve pairs of cranial nerves are largely specialised in their function Numbers 1, 2, 8 and 9 subserve the functions of smell, sight, hearing and taste. respectively. Numbers 3, 4, 6, 7, 11 and 12 are largely motor nerves and the 5th is the sensory nerve of the face. The 10th nerve, or *vagus*, is almost entirely a part of the parasympathetic nervous system, and it has both motor and sensory fibres. These cranial nerves have internal connections of the most complicated nature and it is unnecessary for the present purpose to describe them further.

SECTION 6—MUSCULAR ACTION

The Properties of Muscle

Voluntary muscle as already mentioned, is made up of many muscle bundles, each containing a large number of muscle fibres. The manner in which these fibres receive their nerve supply is shown in Figure 116. Each nerve fibre ends in a small expansion called an *end plate*, which is the terminal portion of the nerve and the part through which the stimulus to contract is given to the muscle fibre. When a muscle fibre contracts it becomes wider and the transverse stripes are drawn closer together (Figure 117, B). When it relaxes, the fibre becomes narrower and the interval between each transverse stripe is increased.

Muscle cannot be compared with an elastic substance because the latter cannot exert a steady pull with accompanying alteration of its length. In many respects muscle action may be compared with the behaviour of the earthworm; when a worm is touched (mechanical stimulus) it contracts, and when the stimulus is removed, it relaxes again. The contractile properties of muscle will be better understood if a practical experiment is described.

The gastrocnemius muscle of a freshly killed frog is dissected out with its nerve supply and fixed on a special stage (Figure 118) with the tendon of the muscle attached to the arm of a lever, which records movements on a slowly revolving drum covered with smoked paper. The nerve is placed across the terminals of an electric machine, capable of emitting a small intermittent current. The current is switched on and off automatically by a special device which can be set to give any required number of electric shocks per second. The recording on this drum in the diagram shows the response of a muscle to a single shock (see also Figure 119, A).

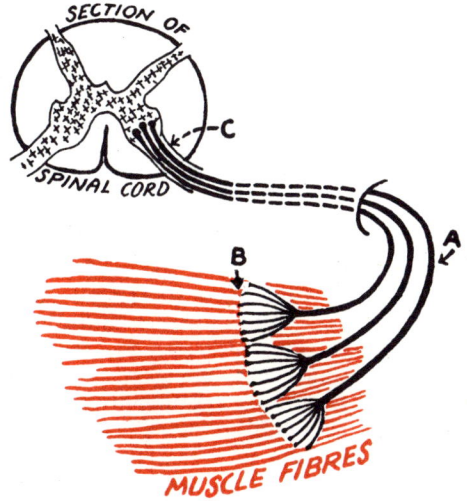

FIGURE 116—Diagram of voluntary or striped muscle fibres with their nerve supply
A—Motor nerve fibre
B—Branches of nerve fibre supplying individual muscle fibres (striping of muscle not shown)
C—Motor nerve fibres leaving anterior horn cells in the grey matter in the spinal cord

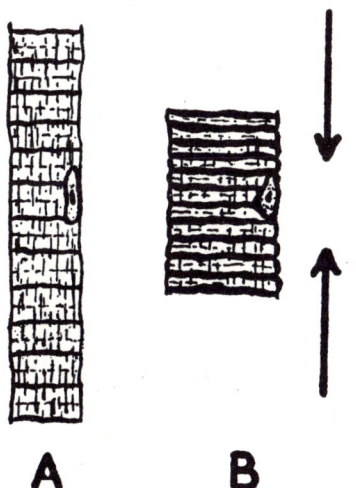

FIGURE 117—Contraction of muscle fibres (diagrammatic)
A—Muscle fibre relaxed
B—Muscle fibre contracted

The responses of the muscle to shocks of varying frequencies are shown in Figure 119. Where frequencies of 20 and 40 shocks per second were employed, the individual results of each shock can be seen as waves in the recorded lines; but the record of the shocks given at 60 per second is a curved line without undulations. This means that at a rate of 60 shocks per second the muscle is unable to relax after one shock before it is stimulated by the next shock, and so it maintains a state of contraction until it is fatigued. In this experiment the voltage of the current remained the same, and so it is clear that the higher frequency of the shocks was responsible for the increase in the pull exerted by the muscle.

In the body, individual fibres of the nerve to a muscle are carrying impulses from the cells in the anterior grey matter of the cord to the muscle fibres which they supply. The activity of the muscle is determined by the total number of these impulses per unit of time. Each anterior horn cell (Figure 116) under the control of the higher nervous centres, sends out its impulses irrespective of what its neighbours are doing. The sum total of all the impulses is reflected in the state of contraction of the muscle. A maximum contraction of the muscle is achieved by a discharge of impulses of all the anterior horn cells which govern the activity of that muscle.

Chemical Changes during Muscle Contraction

Very little is known about the chemical reactions by which energy, stored in the muscles, is converted into mechanical energy, causing the muscle fibres to contract; but it is known that certain chemical substances make their appearance in muscle tissue after a period of activity.

Muscle contains about 15 per cent. of protein and a small quantity of glycogen,* fat and phosphorus. If a muscle is stimulated in an atmosphere free from oxygen, the glycogen disappears and lactic acid replaces it; with continued stimulation in the absence of oxygen, the lactic acid accumulates and the muscle becomes more and more fatigued. The presence of oxygen makes possible the removal of the lactic acid; the exact reaction is not known but some may be converted back to glycogen in the muscles. Oxygen, therefore, is in some way necessary for the removal of lactic acid after a period of muscular activity.

During very strenuous exercise, lactic acid is formed in the tissues in amounts far greater than can be immediately disposed of by the available oxygen, and some of it therefore passes into the blood stream, where it no longer embarrasses the action of the muscle.

An oxygen debt to the tissues is thus incurred which must be paid to remove the excess lactic acid. It is well known that the rate and depth of breathing remain above normal for many minutes after strenuous activity has ceased. The large amounts of oxygen taken in are used to dispose of the lactic acid which has been temporarily neutralized by a special chemical reaction in the blood until enough oxygen to remove it has been supplied by the lungs.

Circulatory and Respiratory Changes during Exercise

The oxygen requirements of the muscles are greatly increased during exercise and at the same time carbon dioxide is elaborated by the muscles and excreted rapidly from the lungs. The circulatory and respiratory systems working together, adapt themselves to meet these requirements. The more important changes which take place are as follows.

1. *Circulatory*

(i) There is an increased return of venous blood to the heart owing to the more extensive movements of the diaphragm and the general contractions of the muscles compressing the veins.

* Glycogen is a carbohydrate which is readily convertible into energy; it is manufactured in the body.

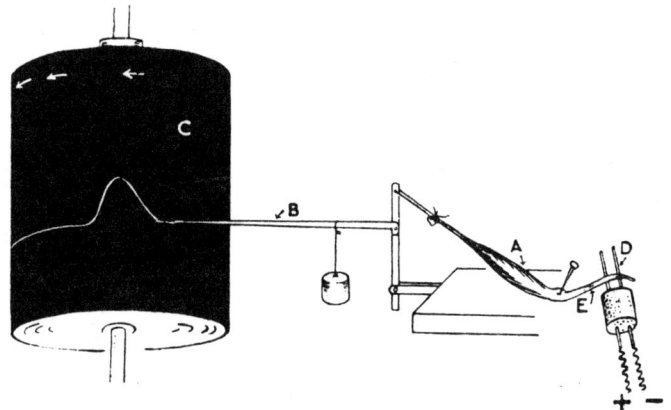

FIGURE 118—Experimental method of recording graphically the response of muscle to small electric shocks

A—Muscle
B—Arm of lever
C—Slowly revolving drum
D—Terminals through which electric stimulus passes
E—Nerve supplying the muscle

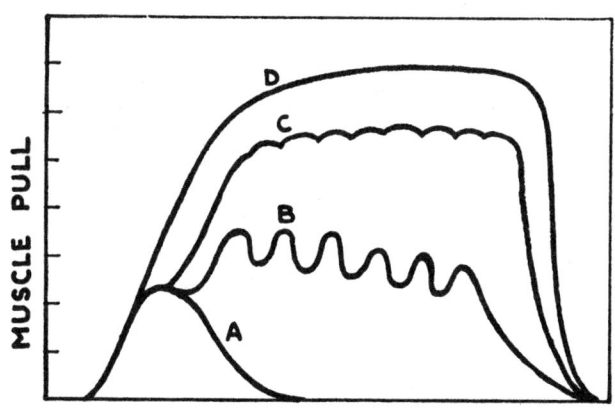

FIGURE 119—A recording of muscle response to shocks of varying frequencies

A—Response to single stimulus
B—Response to 20 stimuli per second
C—Response to 40 stimuli per second
D—Response to 60 stimuli per second

(ii) The rate and output of the heart per beat increase so that a greater volume of blood is circulated per unit of time.

(iii) There is a redistribution of blood; more goes to the muscles and less to the intestines and skin. During exercise a muscle may receive as much as fifteen times its normal flow of blood.

2. *Respiratory*

Respiration becomes much deeper and more rapid; this is mainly brought about by the increase of carbon dioxide in the blood which has an accelerator action on the nervous centre which controls the rate of breathing. This property of carbon dioxide is made use of in anaesthetics; it is given with the anaesthetic and causes the patient to inhale deeply, and reach the required stage of anæsthesia more rapidly.

CHAPTER III

POSTURE AND CORRECTIVE EXERCISES

The development of the fully erect posture is a comparatively recent acquisition of man during his long history of evolution. It must not be regarded in any sense as abnormal, for no development is abnormal which has evolved to suit the mode of life and assist the survival of the particular animal. All such processes of evolution have been brought about naturally; if they were not anatomically or physiologically useful, the animal undergoing them would fail possibly to the point of extinction.

It is impossible to say whether or not the evolution of the erect posture in man is complete; however, the liability of young adults to develop postural defects, sometimes without obvious cause, suggests that the process is not yet entirely finished. The one disadvantage of the erect posture is that the upper limbs, instead of helping to support the forepart of the body, have themselves to be supported, the additional weight being borne by the upper part of the trunk; in consequence there is a tendency for respiratory movements to be hindered if the muscles supporting the shoulder girdle become weakened thereby allowing it to hang forwards and throw its weight upon the walls of the thorax.

The Muscles of Posture (Figure 120)

The muscles of posture are situated mainly on the anterior and posterior aspects of the body.

It is necessary to realize that all the muscles involved in maintaining the erect posture take their fixed points from below and endeavour to balance one bone upon another (Figure 121). The muscles of the foot steady the arch to form a firm basis; the muscles in front of and behind the tibia, steady the tibia on the foot; the femur is balanced on the tibia by the quadriceps in front and the gastrocnemius behind; the position of the pelvis is fixed by the abdominal muscles, the rectus femoris (part of the quadriceps), the psoas, iliacus and by the sartorius, all of which act on the front of the pelvis, and by the gluteus maximus and hamstring muscles, which exert their pull on the back of the pelvis; the gluteus medius, gluteus minimus and tensor fasciae latae prevent the pelvis from tilting sideways; the vertebral column is balanced upon the steady pelvic base by the extensor muscles of the spine, the muscles of the abdominal wall and the muscles of the neck.

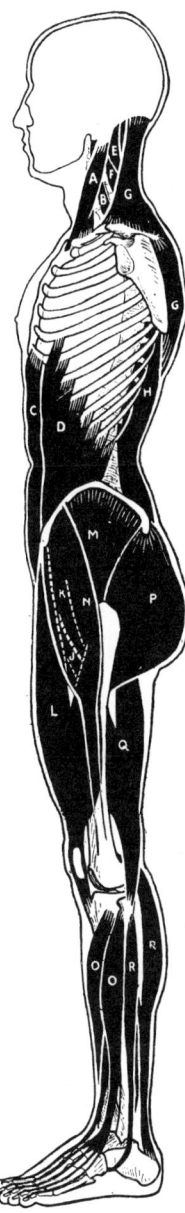

Figure 120—The muscles* which maintain the upright position

(1) *Muscles of the trunk*

(i) Anterior:
   (A) sternomastoid
   (B) longus colli
   (C) rectus abdominis
   (D) oblique muscles of the abdomen

(ii) Posterior:
   (E) splenius capitis
   (F) splenius cervicis
   (G) trapezius
   (H) lower part of long spinal muscles

(2) *Muscles of the lower limb*

(i) Anterior:
   (J) psoas
   (K) iliacus
   (L) quadriceps
   (M) gluteus medius and minimus
   (N) tensor fasciae latae
   (O) long extensors of toes and the anterior tibial muscle

(ii) Posterior:
   (P) gluteus maximus
   (Q) hamstring muscles
   (R) long flexors of toes, the calf and posterior tibial muscle

* Of one side only.

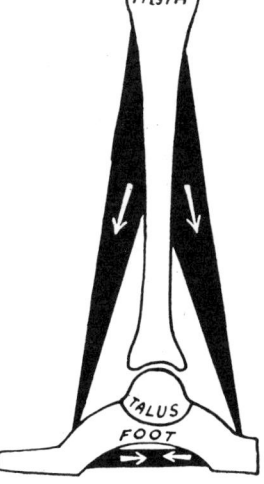

Figure 121—Diagram of muscles of posture acting from fixed point below

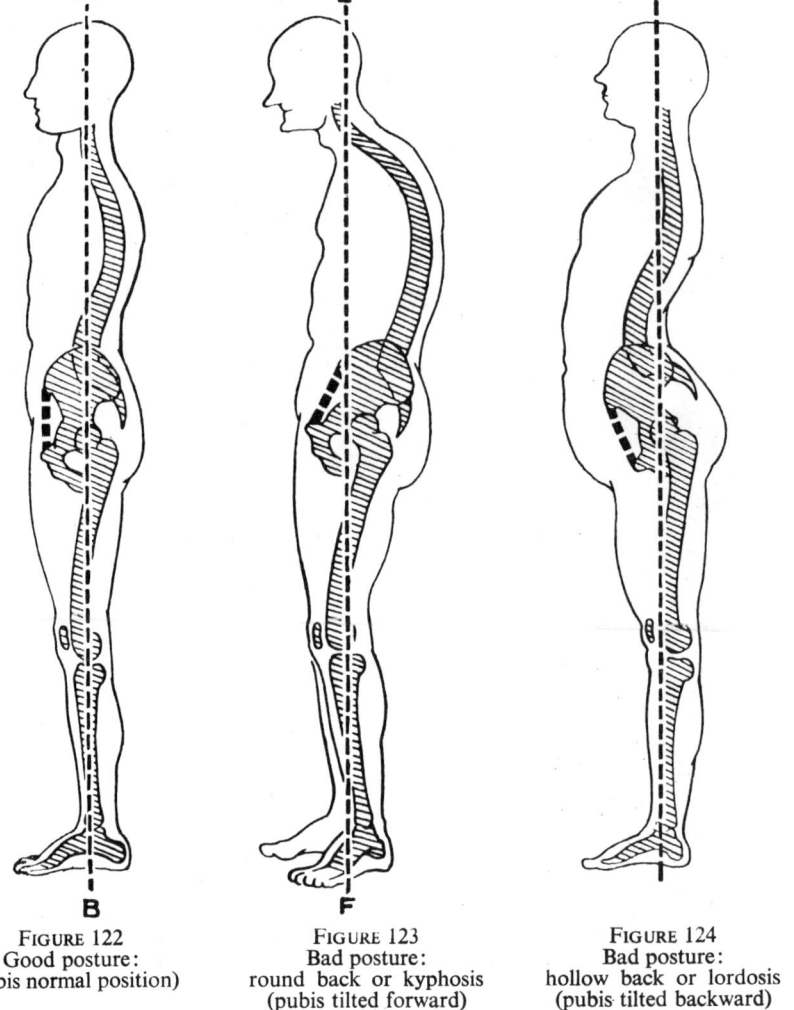

FIGURE 122
Good posture:
(pubis normal position)

FIGURE 123
Bad posture:
round back or kyphosis
(pubis tilted forward)

FIGURE 124
Bad posture:
hollow back or lordosis
(pubis tilted backward)

Good Posture

There is not strictly speaking a *normal* posture because, in spite of the fundamental similarity of structure of all human subjects, variations occur in different individuals.

These variations are sufficiently striking to make possible the grouping of individuals into certain types, the characteristic features of each type being remarkably consistent. There are three main kinds of body structure:

(1) The *Mesomorph or Athletic*. The trapezii are strong and prominent, the chest and shoulders broad, and the waist narrow. The trunk and limbs are muscular, with little fat.

(2) The *Endomorph or Pyknic*. The neck is short and thick; the shoulders are strong but of more graceful construction and more rounded than those of the athletic type. The head, chest and abdomen are massive. The face, trunk and limbs are well covered with fat.

(3) The *Ectomorph or Asthenic*. The neck, trunk and limbs are long and thin, and the chest is long, narrow and flat with prominent ribs. The musculature is generally slight with only a small covering of fat. The joints are small and the profile angular.

The body structures of many people conform fairly exactly to one of these types, but there are many more who combine the features of one type with those of another.

These variations and combinations are of considerable interest to the physical training instructor because they illustrate certain common postural habits, and to the psychiatrist also, because mental characteristics are associated with bodily configuration and posture.

The ideal posture is shown in Figure 122 where the skeleton is held erect in a position mechanically most favourable for the transmission of body weight. The line AB is the perpendicular upon which lies the centre of gravity of the body. The line passes from the highest point of the skull through the weight-bearing surfaces of the cervical and lumbar vertebrae, and through the centres of the hip, knee and ankle joints; the only weight-bearing surfaces through which it does not pass are those of the dorsal vertebrae, owing to the natural curve in that region. This fact is of some importance because the weight of the body above the dorsal region tends to tilt the dorsal vertebrae as shown in Figure 125, the weight being concentrated on the fronts of the bodies, as indicated by the small arrows. In good posture, the minimum contraction of all muscle groups is required to achieve balance. If muscle A is stretched by the tilt of the dorsal vertebrae, muscle contraction is initiated or increased to restore the normal position. Constant stretching of the muscle, and therefore constant contraction of the muscle, causes fatigue in that muscle. Soon this muscle responds by adapting itself to work from this fresh stretched position and triggers off a faulty posture pattern.

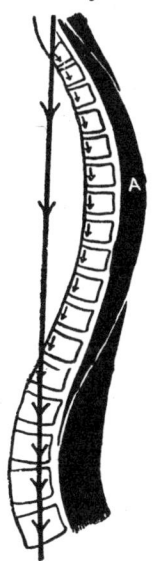

FIGURE 125—Diagram showing the weight distribution in the dorsal and lumbar portion of the normal vertebral column
A—Dorsal part of long spinal muscles

Bad Posture

There are several types of defective posture which give rise to abnormal curvatures in the vertebral column; they are:

(1) The *round* back of *kyphosis* as seen in Figure 123. This defect is invariably accompanied by round shoulders.

(2) The *hollow* back or *lordosis* as seen in Figure 124. The shoulders are held back.

(3) The *round* and *hollow* back combined. The shoulders are usually held forward.

(4) The *rigid spine*. The vertebral column is rigid and its normal curvature in the dorsal region is absent; the shoulders are held forward.

(5) *Scoliosis*. The vertebral column is bent laterally.

1. **Round Back** (Figures 123 and 127)

Figure 123 represents the attitude of the body when there is an increased dorsal curvature. The head is held in a forward position. To adjust the balance, the pubis is tilted forwards, the knees are held slightly flexed and inwardly rotated and the feet are turned outward to an abnormal degree and are placed on a broader base.

The perpendicular EF in Figure 123 does not pass through any of the important weight-bearing surfaces except the knee joint. A result is that an increased strain is thrown upon the extensor muscles and ligaments of the upper part of the spine; in addition the body weight is thrown on to the forepart of the foot instead of being distributed evenly between the heel and the toes. This maldistribution of weight leads to foot strain.

Causes of Round Back

Defective posture under conditions of civilization, is unfortunately very common in apparently normal and healthy people and for this reason the subject must be described in some detail.

The position of the head is very often the influencing factor. This point can be simply illustrated by attaching a brick A, representing the head, on the top of a pile of smaller bricks, in the manner shown in Figure 126, so that it just balances. If A is moved still further forward and all the bricks are attached

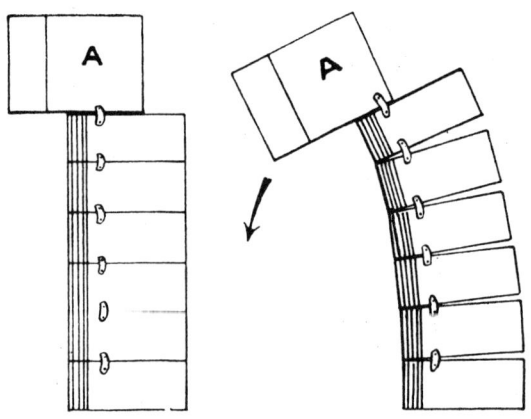

FIGURE 126—Diagram to illustrate the influence of the position of the head upon the vertebral column

to one another, the whole column will curve forward and fall. In the same way the head, being a relatively heavy part of the body, can exert considerable leverage on the upper portion of the vertebral column; the further forward it is held, the greater the strain on the muscles of the neck and upper part of the back. Soon the muscles become fatigued by stretching and the bodily attitude becomes similar to that shown in Figure 123. The forward droop of the shoulders makes the round back appear even worse than it is.

The primary causes of round back and its associated defects of posture are numerous; they include defective vision or hearing, faulty seating arrangements, poor ventilation, poor lighting, overwork and lack of proper exercise, unsuitable clothing, over-rapid growth, and debilitating illnesses. The secondary cause is loss of neuromuscular balance. This type of defect usually develops during the years of growth, particularly between the ages of ten and twenty.

The extent to which vision can influence the position of the head can be seen in children or young adults who have bad sight or incorrect spectacles; they adopt a peering attitude when standing and lean right forward over their books when reading. Further bad habits such as looking over the tops of the spectacles are sometimes developed. Deaf people often acquire the habit of craning their necks forward to assist their hearing. Continuous use of the eyes when studying, in addition to faulty seating arrangements, produces strain of the extensor muscles of the neck and spine.

Tight or rough-edged collars or mufflers worn under an overcoat which restrict head movements may be responsible for the development of faulty carriage of the head. Hats worn on the back of the head may have the same effect. Women often acquire the habit of holding their chins in the air, hoping thereby to avoid the development of a double chin.* Children who grow rapidly are very prone to develop a round back unless a good posture habit is maintained and encouraged.

All illnesses, a part of whose treatment is rest in bed for a long time, produce a general weakness in all body musculature. The young are particularly affected and unless due precautions are taken when the child goes back to school, postural abnormality is likely to develop after sitting for long periods over a desk.

The foundations of good posture are laid during the years of growth, from birth to the age of twenty. If, during this time, certain common-sense principles are followed, development should take a normal course; but if bad habits are formed, a defective posture develops which becomes permanent and more exaggerated as age advances, unless steps are taken to control it by properly planned exercises, games and hobbies.

It is unfortunate that by the time an individual has become interested in posture, it is usually too late to effect a radical improvement. A defect in posture can only be corrected by the individual who suffers from it and, as he usually feels no pain, he often does not make any real effort to carry out the constant parental orders to correct his posture.

All too often the fault lies not with the child but with the parents or those in charge at his place of education or work. In this competitive age of examinations health is sometimes sacrificed for diplomas and certificates; a timely visit to the doctor may be the means of saving the child from having a permanently defective posture.

There are certain diseases which directly affect the bony skeleton and cause curvature of the spine, but these do not come within the scope of this book.

The Principles of Postural Re-education for Round Back and its Associated Defects

The value of postural re-education is greatest during the years of growth. Postural defects which have led to bony or ligamentous changes cannot be cured. Postural re-education may improve those in which there is alteration of the good posture definition (*i.e.* minimum activity of all muscle groups to

---

* In fact, this is one of the best methods of acquiring it, for the tissues under the chin become stretched.

achieve balance). It is essential that medical advice is obtained in every case before any attempt to correct the deformity by postural re-education is made. The aim of this re-education should be to restore the muscular balance and to mobilize joints within normal limits.

Muscles which have become used to working around a fresh rest position following constant stretch must be worked within their normal middle ranges so that the muscles may be able to re-adapt themselves to the correct rest position. It must be remembered that the antagonist has become used to a different rest position and this also requires re-education. Constant use of a muscle in either the inner or outer ranges will lead to the muscle developing a fresh rest position in the middle of the constantly used range.

When instructing an individual with a round back and its associated postural defects, special attention must be paid to the following points:

(i) The position of the head, the round back and shoulders.

(ii) The tilt of the pubis.

(iii) The maldistribution of weight upon the feet.

(i) The head carriage and the round back may be improved by exercises to shorten the extensor muscles of the neck and upper part of the spine, and at the same time lengthen the muscles which bend the neck forwards; that is, to bring them to their mid-range for a good posture definition. These exercises are best carried out lying on the back to eliminate the effect of gravity; a cushion or sandbag should be placed between the shoulder blades. When walking, the head should be held in such a position that the eyes are looking forward and slightly above their own level.

The round shoulders may be corrected by exercises to shorten the trapezii, rhomboids and levatores scapulae, and lengthen the pectoralis major and pectoralis minor. Exercises with the back to the wall bars are especially useful for lengthening the pectoral muscles. The type of exercise most valuable to correct round shoulders is precisely the movement which we almost unconsciously carry out when, after sitting at a desk for some time, we lean back on the chair and brace the shoulders backward thus stretching the pectoral muscles and obtaining a great sense of relief.

When the shoulders are braced back the dorsal spine tends to straighten, as shown in Figure 128. If the muscles A, each representing the trapezius and rhomboids of one side, contract, they not only pull the scapulae towards the mid-line posteriorly but also tend to push the dorsal part of the vertebral column forward in the direction of C, thus helping to correct the curvature. The principle of this mechanism may be more clearly understood by reference to the inset; if the two ends of a string, supporting a weight W, are pulled simultaneously, the weight moves upwards in the direction of X. As the shoulder girdle droops forward so it tends to exaggerate the dorsal kyphosis and add to the stretch on the dorsal muscles.

The position of the shoulder girdle also has a considerable influence on respiration; normally, in a person of good posture, a great deal of the weight of the upper limb is supported by the trapezius and rhomboids, but if the shoulders are allowed to hang forward, they compress the ribs by their weight and hinder proper respiration. Breathing exercises are therefore important in these cases.

(ii) To correct the tilt of the pelvis (Figure 127) exercises should be designed to shorten the flexors of the hip and extensors of the knee, and lengthen the extensors of the hip. Exercises should be performed with the knees straight and, during the early stages, in the recumbent position.

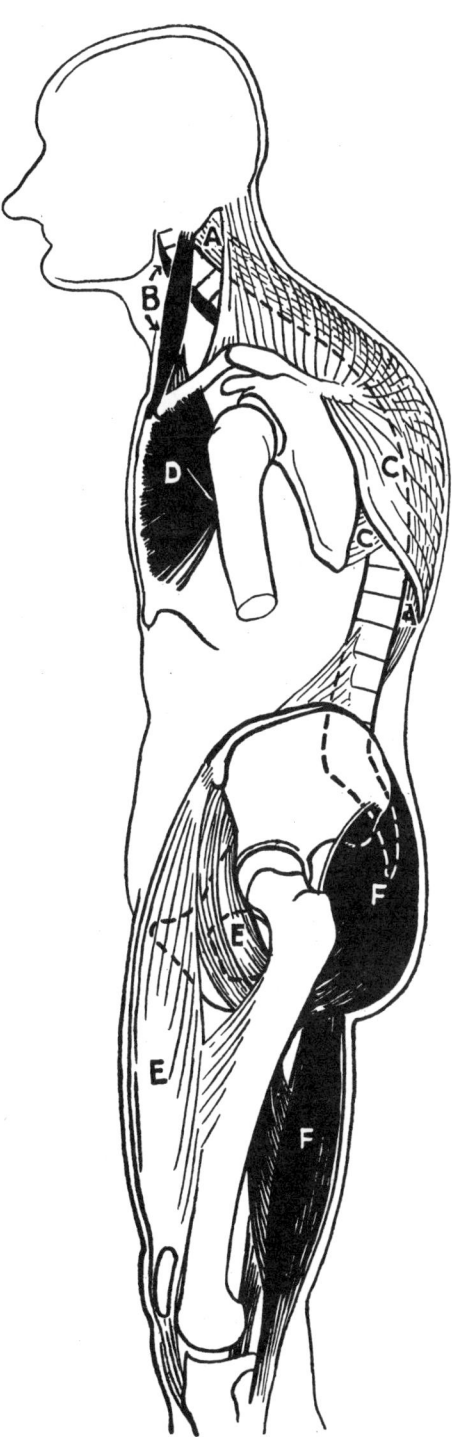

A—Extensors of neck and upper part of back
B—Flexors of the neck
C—Muscles connecting scapula to vertebrae
D—Pectorals
E—Flexors of the hip
F—Extensors of the hip

FIGURE 127—Diagram showing the lengthened muscles (shaded) and the shortened antagonists (black) associated with round back and round shoulders

(iii) The weight-bearing surfaces of normal feet fall along the opposing sides of an imaginary trapezium (Figure 129), the heels being fairly close together and the feet making an angle of approximately 45 degrees with one another; but an individual with a round back usually splays his feet outward because his balance is disturbed. To readjust it, he puts his feet into the positions shown in Figure 130.

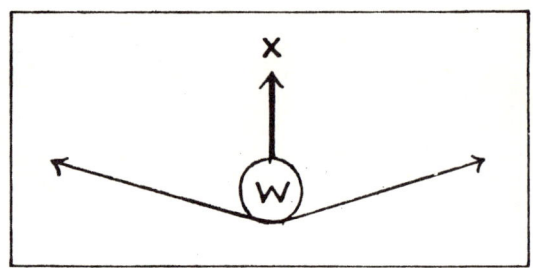

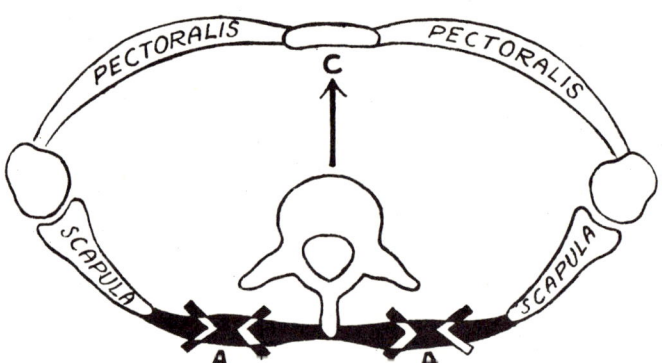

Figure 128—Cross section through dorsal region
A—Trapezius and rhomboids (diagrammatic)

The two arches of the feet placed together should normally form a dome-shaped structure, the roof of the dome being moderately flexible. A foot, in which all the joints are stiff, does not allow the small movements to take place which are necessary to adjust the balance of the body; suppleness and good muscles are essential for the normal functioning of the foot. Negroes have excellent feet; the arches are exceptionally supple and are flattened by weight or raised by powerful foot muscles according to circumstances.

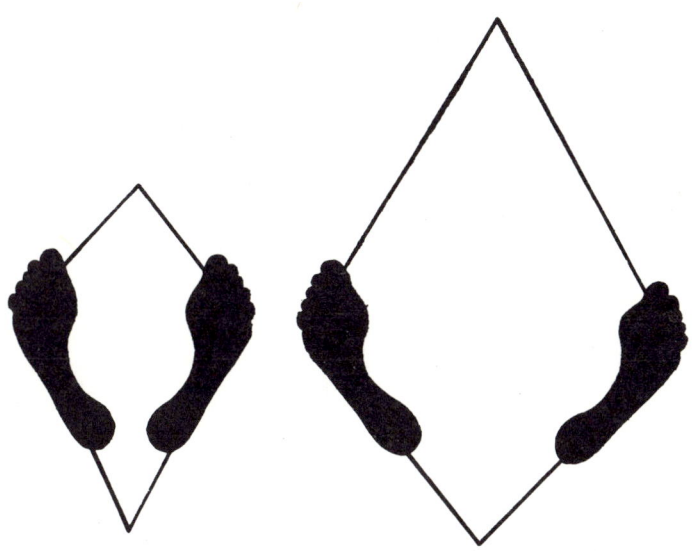

FIGURE 129—Normal position of feet

FIGURE 130—Position of feet when posture is defective

2. The Hollow Back or Lordosis (Figures 124 and 131)

Exaggeration of the lumbar curve is a common defect of posture especially when it is the result of a misguided attempt at maintaining normal posture in the thoracic region.

This leads to the protruding abdomen, the pelvis tilted forward and the knees hyperextended. The effect of gravity on the abdominal contents exaggerates the lordosis and restricts the normal breathing mechanism.

Postural Re-education for Hollow Back

The object of the re-education should be to lengthen the long spinal muscles and the flexors of the hip, and to shorten the abdominal and hamstring muscles. This corrects the pelvic tilt and lumbar scoliosis and restores the correct position for the least activity of muscle groups on either side of the weight-bearing bony surfaces. The following types of exercise should be given:

(i) Flexion of the vertebral column when lying down by moving the trunk upward to the sitting position, the knees must be kept bent to avoid stretching the hamstring muscles; this exercise shortens the recti abdominis, and lengthens the long spinal muscles.

(ii) Rotation of the lower part of the trunk from side to side when lying down with knees bent; this shortens the oblique muscles of the abdomen.

(iii) Extension of the hip with bent knee when lying face downwards; this exercise shortens the hamstring muscles and the glutaeus maximus.

(iv) Pressing the hollow of the back against a flat surface.

(v) Breathing exercises to redevelop the abdominal muscles, particularly the transverse muscles.

It should also be emphasized that where there is overweight associated with this postural pattern, the person should attempt to reduce this after consulting the medical officer.

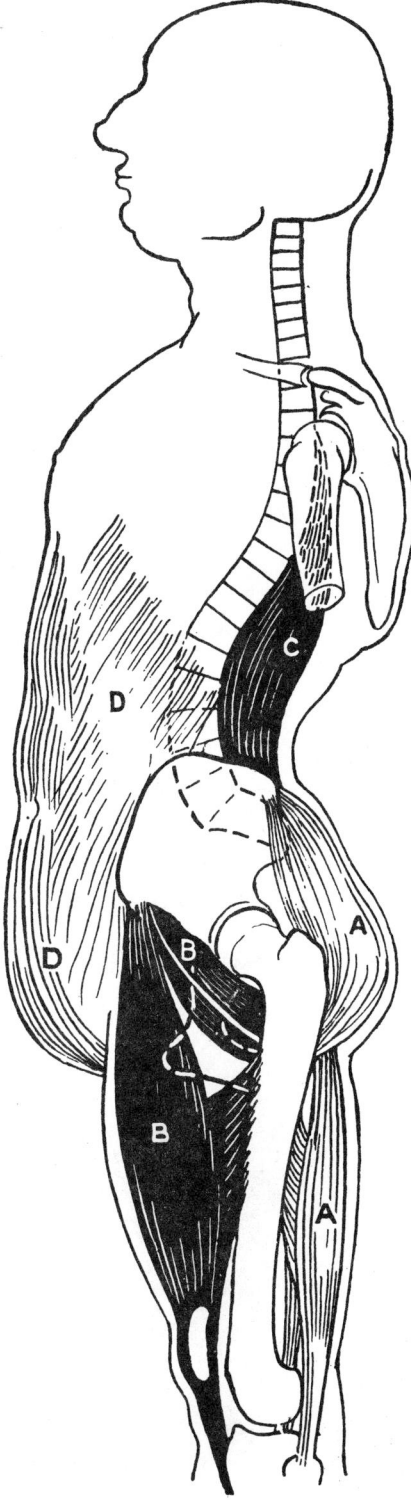

FIGURE 131—Diagram showing the lengthened muscles (shaded) and the shortened antagonists (black) associated with hollow back

  A—Extensors of the hip
  B—Flexors of the hip
  C—Lower portion of long spinal muscles
  D—Muscles of the abdominal wall

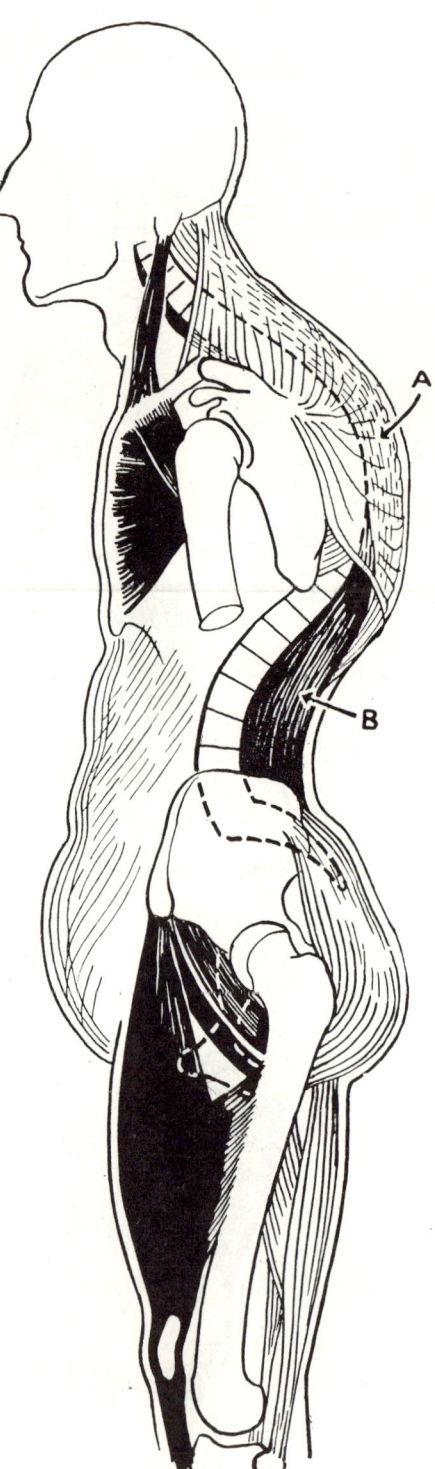

FIGURE 132—Diagram of lengthened muscles (shaded) and shortened antagonists (black) associated with round back and hollow back combined

A—Upper portion of long spinal muscles
B—Lower portion of long spinal muscles

3. Round Back and Hollow Back Combined (Figure 132)

These two postural defects are sometimes present together. The exercises outlined above for round back and hollow back are applicable, but special attention should be paid to the spinal muscles, because the upper portions are elongated and the lower portions are shortened. Exercises should therefore be given chiefly lying down, when the effect of gravity is removed and the action of the spinal muscles can be more easily isolated.

4. Rigid Spine

This is the name for a back which has lost its normal flexibility and in which the musculature is little used; movement is restricted chiefly in the lower dorsal and upper lumbar regions. This type of defect is present in a very large number of people, particularly in those who are accustomed to lead a sedentary life and who never take exercise. It is often associated with round shoulders owing to shortening of the pectoral muscles; the back, however, is usually straighter than normal.

The defect may be corrected or improved, according to the extent of the rigidity present, by simple trunk bending exercises in which particular attention is paid to rotation of the trunk; exercises for breathing and general co-ordination are essential. Here the accent is on mobilization of joints.

5. Lateral Curvature of the Spine or Scoliosis

There may be one large C-shaped curve extending the whole length of the spine (Figure 133, A) or two smaller curves, one the primary B, the other the compensatory curve D.

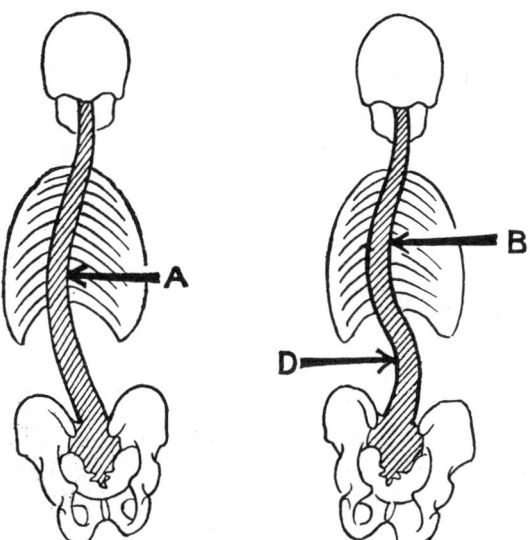

FIGURE 133—Types of scoliosis (diagrammatic)
A—Single C-shaped curve   B—Primary curve
D—Compensatory curve

The causes of scoliosis are numerous; it is frequently the first sign of some underlying disease or injury and medical advice should always be obtained before any attempt is made to correct the deformity by exercise.

The type of scoliosis which can be corrected by exercise is postural in origin and usually consists of a single C-shaped curve; in the majority of cases it is directed to the left, because the majority of people are right-handed and the weight of the elevated arm tilts the spine slightly towards the opposite side of

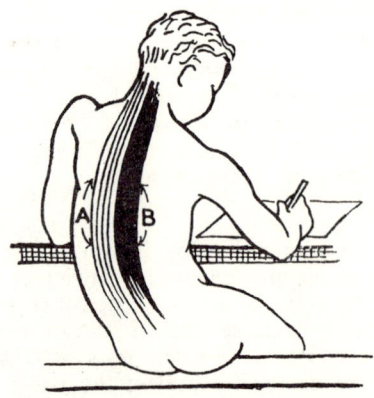

FIGURE 134—A faulty sitting position which may cause scoliosis
A—Lengthened long and spinal muscles
B—Shortened long spinal muscles

the body. When a person carries a bucket of water in his right hand, he usually raises his left arm to act as a counterweight. Postural scoliosis is often caused through faulty habits when working at a table or desk (Figure 134). It is associated with round back, round shoulders, and weakness of the muscles supporting the arches of the feet. The ilium on the side of the convexity is rotated forward and on the opposite side it is rotated backward.

Postural scoliosis is caused by a muscular imbalance between muscles which have the same primary action. The long muscles of the spine on the side of the convexity become longer than those in the opposite side; exercise should therefore aim at shortening the former and lengthening the latter, but general exercises are equally important to maintain mobility.

The type of case which is likely to respond well to exercise is the one in which the scoliosis disappears when the spine is flexed.

Corrective Exercise for Scoliosis

The following types of exercise are recommended.

(i) General spinal exercises; flexion, extension, rotation and lateral flexion.

(ii) Beam hanging with lateral flexion, particularly towards the side of the convexity. All forms of hanging exercises help to straighten the spine.

(iii) By a process of trial and error, the individual can usually eliminate the scoliosis by manoeuvring his shoulders and arms into a certain position; if, for example, the scoliosis has a convexity to the left it may be corrected by the contraction of the trapezius, rhomboids and latissimus dorsi on the right side, and the relaxation of the same muscles on the left side. These muscles, being attached to the spines of the dorsal vertebrae, can, when contracting unilaterally, exert a considerable influence on the position of the spine. Having once found the position which causes the scoliosis to disappear, the individual should be encouraged to become used to this new posture pattern by constant practice in front of a mirror.

(iv) Breathing and general co-ordination exercises should be given; swimming, using the breast stroke, is most valuable for this and all other types of postural defects.

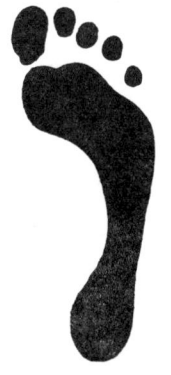 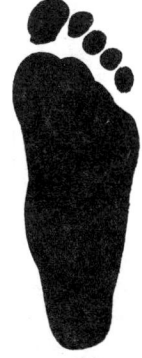

FIGURE 135—Footprint of normal foot   FIGURE 136—Footprint of flat foot

Defects of the Feet

It is convenient at this point to describe the defects of the feet, which are commonly caused by faulty posture, unsuitable footwear, prolonged standing, excessive body weight, or lack of proper exercise.

There are several types of foot deformity, in addition to ordinary flat foot, which may give rise to pain; of these the stiff foot with the high arch and the foot with the great toe deviated across the second toe, are the most common. Their treatment is largely a medical problem and will not therefore be described.

The painful flat foot is perhaps the commonest type of disability of the feet; in the early stages, before the foot has lost flexibility in the joints, it responds to treatment by exercise, although six months of constant exercise may be required to restore the normal muscle pattern effectively and bring about a relief from pain.

As already mentioned, it is the loss of use of the muscles supporting the arch of the foot which produces a flattening of the arch; the bones on the inner border of the arch take up abnormal positions and adhesions form, fixing the bones in a position of deformity. Pain is caused when the ligaments, which are then subjected to abnormal strains, are put on the stretch by weight-bearing. The degree of flattening of an arch may be assessed by examining an active footprint which may be obtained by walking along a smooth, slightly absorbent surface with a wet foot. It is important that the print is one taken during normal walking as many people without weak muscles stand with flat arches and may produce a footprint like that in Figure 136. Figure 135 shows the footprint of a normal foot and Figure 136 that of a markedly flat foot, where the inner border of the arch is in full contact with the ground.

The muscles which support the arches of the foot are the anterior tibial, the posterior tibial, the long flexors of the toes, the peroneus longus and the small muscles of the foot (Figure 137).

Corrective exercises should be given upon the following lines.

(1) Instruction in walking with the feet parallel to one another; also walking on the outer borders of the feet to strengthen the invertors (the anterior and posterior tibial muscles).

(2) Heel and toe walking; the toes should be made to grip the ground.

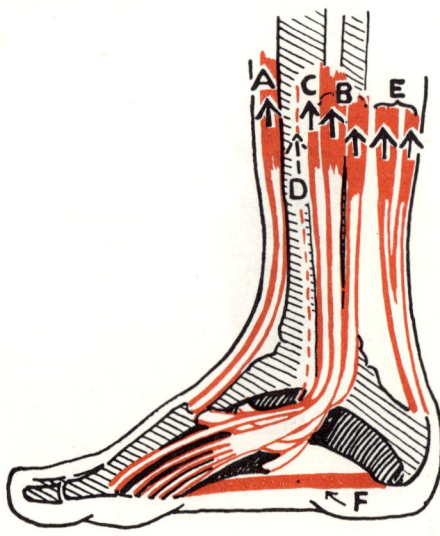

FIGURE 137—Diagram showing the muscles which support the arch of the foot

A—Anterior tibial muscle
B—Long flexors of the toes
C—Posterior tibial muscle
D—Peroneus longus (obscured by the bones)
E—Calf muscles
F—Small muscles of the foot

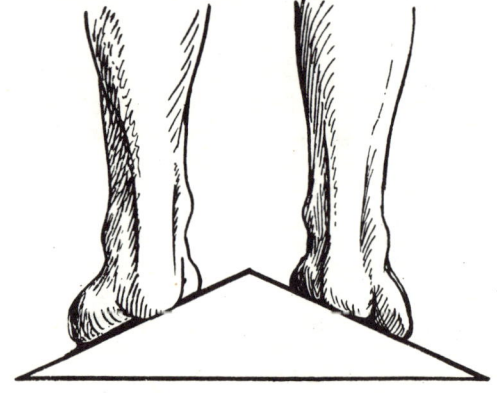

FIGURE 138—Board used for producing inversion

(3) Heel walking; this strengthens the anterior tibial muscles and lengthens the calf muscles (gastrocnemius and soleus).

(4) Walking on sloping surfaces; a triangular board is most useful for this exercise (Figure 138).

(5) Tip-toe exercises with bowed knees, throwing the weight on the outer borders of the foot; backward hopping with knees bent, and later, forward hopping exercises.

(6) Foot-shortening exercises, in which an attempt is made with the weight-bearing foot to shorten and narrow the foot with the toes stretched out and gripping the ground. This raises the heads of the metatarsals in the centre of the foot and also shortens the longitudinal arch, thus raising it. This type of exercise may be difficult to teach but is the most rewarding of all flat foot exercises; it requires a mobile foot in order to be effective as do all the above exercises.

Many types of exercise may be devised on these lines but it is important to bear in mind that any exercise which stretches the small muscles of the foot such as weight-bearing on the everted foot is harmful and delays recovery. The individual should do his exercises with bare feet on a smooth surface; they should be performed either sitting or standing according to the degree of muscle tone present. The type, vigour and duration of exercise should be regulated according to the capacity to complete them without fatigue. This principle applies to the giving of every type of exercise, particularly corrective exercises for painful flat feet.

CHAPTER IV

BREATHING

THE rhythmical movements of respiration are under the control of a centre in the lower part of the brain called the *respiratory* centre, from which regular impulses are transmitted to the diaphragm, the intercostal muscles and the abdominal muscles; this centre is in its turn under the control of the cerebrum. Normal respiration is performed without conscious effort, just as posture may be maintained without interference by the cerebrum; conscious effort is made only when we wish to bring about a change in the character of our respiration or to hold our breath.

The respiratory centre discharges impulses rhythmically about 15 times per minute during normal breathing and is responsible for the respiratory rate. The ratio of the pulse rate to the respiratory rate in a healthy man at rest is about four to one.

The Mechanism of Normal Respiration

An account of the structure and function of the respiratory apparatus has already been given in earlier chapters; the various mechanisms of normal breathing will now be described.

Normal respiration may, for the purposes of description, be divided into *quiet* and *deep* respiration; there is no essential difference between the two.

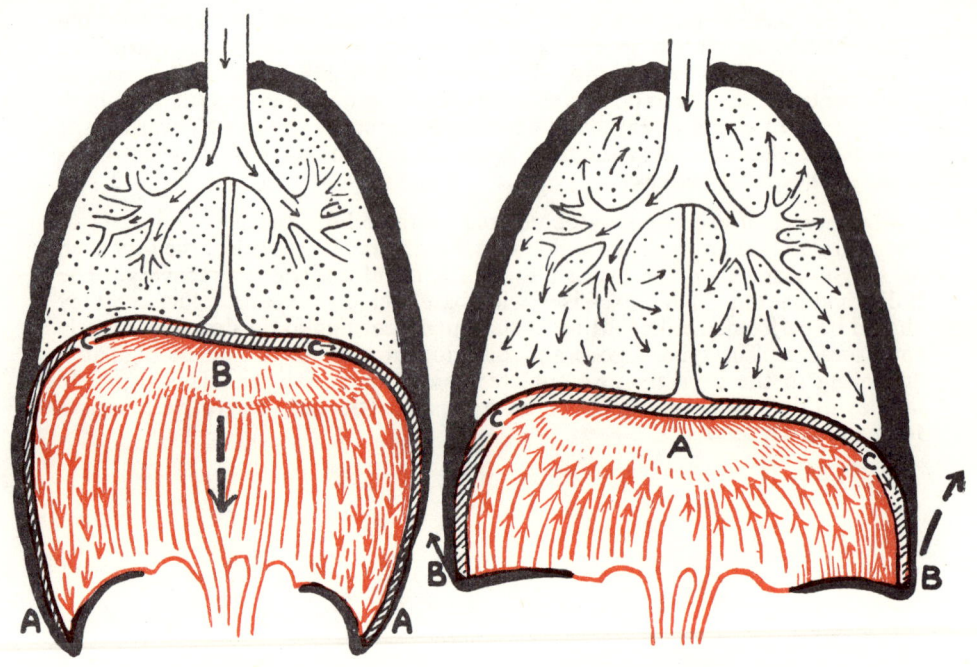

FIGURE 139—Early inspiration
The diaphragm contracting from the ribs as fixed point
A—Lower ribs
B—Diaphragm moving down
C—Cut edge of diaphragm

FIGURE 140—Late inspiration
The diaphragm contracting from its central tendon as fixed point
A—Diaphragm
B—Lower ribs moving upward and outward

Quiet Respiration (Figures 139 and 140)

Quiet respiration is performed by the diaphragm, the intercostal muscles and the abdominal muscles. At the beginning of inspiration the diaphragm begins to move down taking its fixed point from the lower margins of the ribs (Figure 139) and in so doing draws air into the lungs through the bronchial tubes, and at the same time pushes the abdominal contents before it until the resistance of the abdominal muscles prevents further downward movement; the level reached by the diaphragm depends upon the force of its contraction and the tone of the muscles of the abdominal wall. When this level is reached, the central tendon of the diaphragm becomes the fixed point for its action (Figure 140) and working in conjunction with the intercostal muscles, it lifts the lower ribs which in turn push forward and raise the sternum and upper ribs. The movement of the diaphragm in Figures 139 and 140 has been exaggerated, the actual range in quiet respiration being abouth three-quarters of an inch with very little alteration of diaphragmatic shape.

The abdominal muscles adjust their tone in relation to the pressure within the abdominal cavity; they are therefore in a state of greater tone at the end of inspiration than at the beginning.

Expiration is effected by the elastic recoil of the thoracic walls assisted by the action of the abdominal muscles which push back the displaced viscera and pull down the sternum.

Deep Respiration

The mechanism of deep inspiration is the same as that of quiet inspiration with additional muscular help to produce an increased expansion of the thorax. The head, neck and upper part of the trunk are extended to enable the sternomastoid and scalene muscles to act on the sternum and upper ribs; the shoulder girdle is braced back so that the pectoral muscles can raise the ribs sideways; and in addition the trapezii help indirectly to expand the thorax by taking the weight of the shoulder girdle off the chest wall. The latissimi dorsi and quadrati lumborum fix the lower ribs, enabling the diaphragm to make stronger and more extensive movements. During forcible expiration, all the muscles of the abdominal wall contract strongly.

Varieties of Breathing

Normal respiration involves a well balanced use of the diaphragm, the thoracic muscles and the abdominal muscles. There are certain people who as a result of habit, disease or injury, use the thoracic muscles predominantly, neglecting the diaphragm and abdominal muscles and vice versa; for this reason there are said to be *diaphragmatic* and *thoracic* types of breathing.

It is perfectly natural under certain conditions to use one or other type of breathing, only for short periods, but the continuous use of one leads to the inefficient working of the other. The ability to breathe by either of these methods safeguards the proper functioning of respiration, and enables us to obtain the necessary oxygen by using one type of breathing only if the other happens to be temporarily restricted. Persons with poor chest expansion commonly suffer from associated pathological conditions, of a mild, chronic type, in their air passages and lungs. Abdominal operations on such persons, who are mainly diaphragmatic breathers, may therefore be complicated by pneumonia because respiratory movements after recovery from the anaesthetic are restricted by the pain in the abdominal wall, and the chest expansion is not great enough to provide adequate ventilation of the lungs. It is interesting to note that babies breathe entirely with their diaphragms; the shape of a baby's chest is circular (Figure 141) and therefore allows no increase in size; but the adult shape is oval, allowing increase in its cross-sectional area. Pneumonia is one of the more common fatal complications of illnesses in babies because the full function of their respiratory apparatus has not been developed.

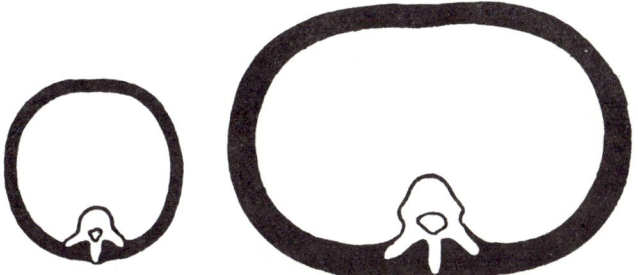

FIGURE 141—Shape of baby's chest

FIGURE 142—Shape of adult's chest (cross-section)

The size and degree of expansion of a person's chest is no indication of correct and well balanced breathing. The size of the chest may be very misleading, in fact a large barrel-shaped chest is often rigid, having lost its elastic recoil and the breathing is almost entirely diaphragmatic, assisted by a heaving movement of the whole thorax at times of exertion. Persons possessing this type of chest frequently suffer from chronic respiratory infections, such as bronchitis.

The idea that diaphragmatic breathing causes weakening of the abdominal wall is quite erroneous; on the contrary, the abdominal muscles are strengthened in accordance with the principle that the more work a muscle performs, the stronger it becomes, provided, of course, it is worked within its capacity.

Factors which cause too great a dependence on the diaphragm are as follows.
(1) Habit.
(2) Bad posture; round back and shoulders as mentioned above, restrict the normal entry of air into the lungs, and cause a shallow type of breathing.
(3) Tight clothing or strapping worn round the chest; web equipment does not restrict chest movement as much as would be expected, because the straps pass over and under each shoulder, thus helping to brace back the shoulder girdles.

Factors giving rise to thoracic breathing are as follows.
(1) Habits of mind* or of body.
(2) Weak abdominal musculature, as may be found in a person with a hollow back.
(3) Tight clothing which restricts, and therefore weakens the normal action of the abdominal muscles. This applies more particulary to women who wear tight corsets. A century ago female clothing was deliberately designed to produce thoracic breathing because it was considered not unattractive.

Normal respiration should be a combination of diaphragmatic and thoracic breathing; both systems are thereby kept in good working order and enable the respiratory apparatus to function at its maximum efficiency.

Deep Breathing Exercises

The purposes of breathing exercises are to increase the mobility of the chest wall, develop the power of muscles concerned with respiration and improve their co-ordination, correct any faults which may be present, and rid the lungs of stale air and refill them with fresh air. Breathing exercises are not effective unless the lungs are filled and emptied to their maximum with each inspiration and expiration; for this reason the term deep breathing has been used above. Such exercises correctly taught and intelligently performed can produce a marked improvement in general health and raise resistance to infection in persons who have developed bad breathing habits; they also increase the capacity for exercise. Ordinary physical activities certainly improve the efficiency of the respiratory system but are usually not enough to correct and control bad habits in breathing.

The following points should be borne in mind in conducting deep breathing exercises.

(1) All deep breathing exercises should be done out-of-doors; if this is not possible, all the windows of the gymnasium or room must be widely opened. It is a great mistake to instruct a class to perform deep breathing exercises after a period of vigorous exercises in a gymnasium with the windows shut, when all the dust has been thoroughly stirred; the muscles of respiration may obtain some benefit but the lungs are filled with dust particles, bacteria and stale air, which more than counteracts any good effect which may be achieved.

(2) Breathing exercises should not be done by numbers, for the vital capacities of different individuals vary widely and therefore the times taken to fill and empty the lungs also vary. Exercises should be carried out in the person's own time; at least ten seconds are needed for inhalation and exhalation and a rest of a few seconds should always be taken between each breath otherwise a sensation of giddiness may be produced. This is a perfectly natural and harmless sequel to over-ventilation of the lungs but it is advisable to avoid it if possible.

(3) There is no definite rule about the best time during the physical training period when breathing exercises should be given; the decision should be left to the instructor. Generally speaking the best time is immediately after a

---

* The emotions have a great effect on bodily states; the circulatory, alimentary and respiratory systems are particularly affected. Depression influences posture in an easily recognized way; the shoulders are rounded, the gait is restricted and the respiratory excursion is diminished. Chronic anxiety, but not fear, sometimes causes thoracic breathing with an increase of the respiratory rate.

period of activity but this applies only to a class undergoing general physical training, none of whom require special corrective exercises in breathing. Persons who are confirmed thoracic or diaphragmatic breathers and have associated postural defects, should always be given separate instruction; they find great difficulty in cultivating correct breathing habits if they are included in class activities. Such persons should be introduced to general exercises slowly, first performing only that type of exercise which can be accomplished easily without interfering with breathing.

(4) Breathing exercises are usually performed to the best advantage in the standing position which allows complete freedom of movement for the upper part of the body. The hands should be placed on the hips, so that the weight of the upper limbs is taken on the hips and the pectoral muscles have a fixed point from which to assist in elevating the ribs during inspiration. The feet should be placed apart.

(5) It is frequently taught that air should be inhaled through the nose and exhaled through the mouth. There is no good reason for this and there are two very good reasons why it should not be done; first, the thorough ventilation of the nasal passages is important and can be produced much more efficiency by a two-way current of air, and secondly, it is an unnatural method of breathing.

Those who breathe habitually through their mouths are difficult to cure. The effect of mouth breathing is to draw into the lungs air which has not been heated or filtered as it would have been had it passed through the nasal passages; thus not only do a great many bacteria and dust particles gain access to the bronchial tubes and lungs but the nasal passages become unhealthy and congested as a result of insufficient ventilation. The most the instructor can do is to explain these points to those who adopt this mode of breathing; the cure lies with the patient.

Inspiration (Figure 143)

The head, neck and upper part of the spine are gradually extended enabling the sternomastoid and scalene muscles to assist in raising the sternum and upper ribs. The elbows and shoulder girdle are rotated backward, a movement which helps to straighten the spine and puts the pectoral muscles in a better position for elevating the ribs sideways.* The pull thus exerted by muscles

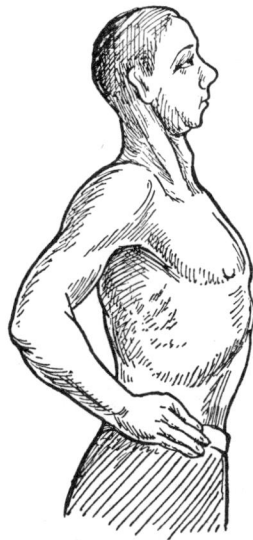
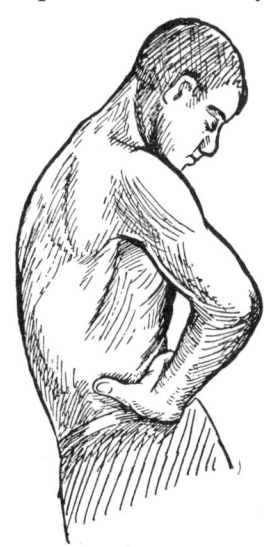

FIGURE 143—The attitude of the body during inspiration

FIGURE 144—The attitude of the body at the end of expiration

* It is mainly for this reason that a boxer rests his arms on the ropes during the interval between the rounds.

outside the thorax provides a fixed point from which the intermediate and lower intercostal muscles can contract to raise the ribs sideways and upward. While inspiration is taking place, the diaphragm is moving down and the tone of the abdominal muscles is increasing in relation to the rise of pressure within the abdominal cavity; the lower intercostals come into full contraction and thus expand and raise the lower part of the thorax at the end of inspiration.

Expiration

During expiration, the head, neck and upper part of the trunk are gradually allowed to flex and the shoulder girdle and elbows are rotated forward; these movements assist the relaxation of the sternomastoid, scalene and pectoral muscles and prevent any interference with the elastic recoil of the ribs. Towards the end of expiration the abdominal muscles are forcibly contracted in order to push up the diaphragm to its maximum extent and so empty the lungs as completely as possible.

There are several other types of breathing exercises but they are not essentially different.

CHAPTER V
FITNESS FOR FLYING

THE various systems of the body not under voluntary control, namely, the circulatory, digestive, nervous, excretory, and to some extent, respiratory, normally perform their functions in an automatic manner, and they require no special attention other than that devoted to keeping the body healthy. On the other hand, the voluntary muscular system does not function normally unless it is exercised, at play, sport or work; muscle thrives on work which is within its capacity to perform, and the tone of muscle is an index of the amount of work performed by it. For example, the blacksmith has abnormally strong arms and shoulder muscles, the old-fashioned postman has strong legs, the jockey has powerful adductors of the legs and the footballer powerful quadriceps. Therefore, we can if we wish, train certain groups of muscles to perform a greater amount of work than is normally required of them.

These considerations are of value to flying personnel, though at first sight it may not appear that flying involves great physical exertion. In fact, during flight, certain muscle groups are used continuously without adequate relaxation, with the result that there is a falling off in efficiency towards the end of the flight owing to muscular discomfort and fatigue; similar discomfort as a result of driving motor cars and lorries is well known. This fatigue can be largely avoided or mitigated and the instructor can help flying personnel by understanding and interpreting its cause.

Muscular Fatigue

Muscular fatigue occurs after a long continued effort or a short intensive physical strain. A long continued effort is the more important, and by virtue of the circumstances of flying, is the common cause of fatigue among flying personnel.

The processes which bring about physical fatigue are but little understood; fatigue after a violent strain may be due to a slight deficiency of oxygen in the arterial blood, which causes a depression of the higher centres in the brain, but during a long continued effort it is possible that products are released by the muscles during their contraction and have a depressant effect upon the central nervous system, reducing its power of sending out nervous impulses. However that may be, it is undoubtedly true that *nervous fatigue*, apart from physical fatigue, generally has an important effect upon behaviour; actions demand greater effort and it is less easy to carry out methodical and complicated tasks. Individuals who are of a nervous temperament suffer more than those who are placid, mostly because their efforts are inefficient. The local discomfort of fatigue is due to an accumulation of exuded fluid between muscle fibres; it causes stiffness and some swelling.

It has already been shown that people are not usually acutely aware of the sensations which arise from the various parts of their limbs; these sensations can exert their effect without the intervention of consciousness, but as fatigue develops sensations become more noticeable and later unpleasant, while the mind at the same time is less tolerant of them. A tired man tends to concentrate his attention on his bodily state and pay increasingly less attention to his behaviour from moment to moment; his capacity for smoothly co-ordinated movement is reduced. Later, in an attempt to avoid the sensations of discomfort he may restrict the attention which he pays both of them and to events in the world about him. These preoccupations may cause failure to notice events of vital importance, for example, an air gunner may fail to see the approach of enemy aircraft or a pilot may fail to check his instruments and carry out his drill with adequate care.

The Relief of Muscular Fatigue when Flying

The only way to relieve discomfort in flight is to increase the circulation, in order to bring more oxygen to the affected parts and help to prevent cramp in the muscles by contracting and relaxing them. The pilot is most likely to feel fatigue in his neck and shoulder muscles from holding his head and upper limbs in one position for a long time. He should extend the neck fully and relax it completely several times, repeating the series of movements at convenient intervals during flight. The aching in the shoulder muscles can be relieved by circular movement of the shoulder girdle, and discomfort in the legs may be overcome by alternate contraction and relaxation of the quadriceps and calf muscles, the chief muscles controlling the rudder bar. Backache may be relieved by full extension and relaxation of the spine. These muscular contractions should be carried out slowly, imitating the natural stretching which occurs almost automatically in people who have been asleep or in the same position for a long time. It is most important that they should be carried out fully as well as slowly, and that they should be repeated an adequate number of times. It is not difficult with a little training, to develop a habit of such movements and there is no doubt that they are even more valuable when performed without the conscious effort of remembering.

Similar movements with appropriate modifications are recommended for other members of aircrew; rear gunners who occupy a cramped position and who have the exacting task of searching the sky for enemies are likely to suffer from backache as well as general muscular discomfort; it is very important that they should take advantage of all opportunities to stretch and relax their muscles.

Mental Fatigue

Mental fatigue is as little understood as physical fatigue, but it is well known that the continuous concentration required during long flights to keep the aircraft on course, and the fear of bad weather, mechanical defects or enemy attack, are potent factors in producing mental fatigue. It is in no way abnormal and is the obvious sequel to a prolonged period of mental strain. It does not harm healthy individuals provided they can obtain enough rest and sleep between operations.

Abdominal Musculature

A good general physique is of great advantage to all flying personnel, and the abdominal muscles are of particular importance to pilots flying fast single-seater aircraft. A strong abdominal musculature can help to prevent *blacking-out*. Blacking-out is a variety of faint caused by a temporary lack of oxygen-carrying blood in the eyes and brain. The forces of gravity and momentum act upon all parts of the body, including the blood, which behave like any other masses, according to the laws of motion. Changes of speed or direction can only be brought about by applying a force to the mass concerned. Changes of direction are particularly important to pilots of fast machines. One of the laws of motion states that a mass at rest continues in a state of rest, and a mass in motion continues to move at the same speed and in the same direction unless forces are brought to bear upon it. An aircraft moving at a high speed has gathered considerable momentum; when the pilot banks the aircraft to make a tight turn, the wing plane becomes almost vertical. The force then applied to the aircraft comes from the pressure of the air beneath the wing surfaces; this is transmitted to the pilot's seat and legs and thence to the rest of his body. The bony framework of the body is not affected but the soft parts, that is, the flesh and organs, strain upon their attachments; the tissues of the face, for example, can be seen to sag and the eyelids to droop. The blood being fluid is particularly affected; it can be acted upon only by the resistance and friction of the blood vessels, which, being elastic, cannot exert a rigid pressure. The blood acting in accordance with this law of motion, continues to travel in the direction in which it was originally travelling until the force exerted by the arteries is sufficient to overcome its momentum. During this period the blood forces its way down into the dependent parts of the body, and the heart, which is attempting to pump it into the head, that is, away from the direction of its original motion, has to deal with a fluid made many times more heavy than its original weight by the momentum which has been imparted to it. A level is reached at which the heart is unable to send enough blood to the brain; first the sensitive retina at the back of the eye ceases temporarily to function and the first stage of blacking-out is reached. If the process continues, consciousness is lost momentarily owing to shortage of oxygen in the brain. Recovery rapidly occurs when the new direction has been achieved and the aircraft has returned to straight flight. The same state of affairs is caused when the aircraft is pulled sharply out of a dive; the blood tries to continue in the direction in which it was previously going, namely forward and downward, while the body of the pilot is forced up by the aircraft. Some estimation of the force applied by the blood can be made by swinging the arm round and round at the shoulder joint as though it were a flail; the hand becomes engorged with blood and if the motion is performed too violently and for too long, small haemorrhages in the skin and beneath the finger nails occur.

    The forces acting on the aircraft, the body, and with it the blood, are expressed in terms of multiples of the force due to gravity designated by the letter g; g is that force which acting upon a mass, causes an acceleration of 32 feet per second per second. Quick changes in direction of an aircraft moving at speed can cause the development of many times this force, which, of course, affects any occupants of the aircraft. Expressed more simply, a force of seven times g —enough to cause blacking-out in the majority of persons—means that the body apparently weighs seven times its normal weight; under these circumstances the blood is as heavy as molten iron and it is easy to see that the heart has considerable difficulty in maintaining the circulation to the head.

    These sensations are readily appreciated during violent manoeuvres in flight; the pilot feels himself being forced down into his seat and he can sense a distension of the lower parts of his body with blood, which accumulates mainly in the legs and abdomen. The amount of g which a man can withstand under these circumstances depends upon his physical health, his physique and the state of his musculature, particularly the abdominal musculature. Good health helps him to counteract the draining away of his blood and the difficulties under which his heart is working; a short, stocky physique makes shorter the distance between the heart and the head and consequently lessens the problem of pumping blood up the vessels to the brain; good firm muscles in the legs have a small action in preventing distension of the vessels of the legs with blood; the abdominal musculature and the diaphragm, by their firm contraction, can squeeze the abdominal contents, raising the intra-abdominal pressure and preventing the blood from pooling within the abdomen. There is no doubt that the last factor particularly has a marked effect in counteracting g. It is of interest to note that legless pilots can withstand a high force exerted by g without blacking-out, because, of course, they have no space in their legs into which the blood can drain.

The importance of preventing blacking-out as far as possible is obvious. In an aerial battle, two pilots in fighter aircraft of comparable performance each trying to shoot the other down, are subject to roughly the same amounts of g. The one who retains vision and consciousness successfully, despite all his manoeuvres, has an enormous advantage over an opponent who suffers even slight effects of g.

There are other methods whereby g can be counteracted, but these are not within the scope of this book.

Practice and exercise in searching the sky for an enemy are also of great value to fighter pilots; tilting the head backward to obtain a better view and particularly turning the extended neck, increase the distance over which the heart must pump blood to the eyes and brain and cause greater arterial resistance Ill effects are reduced by constant exercise.

General Health

Good health is a priceless possession to any man; this must be obvious but it is not always clear how discomforts and dangers can be mitigated by paying attention to maintaining health. Certain problems which all flying personnel meet sooner or later can be solved at least in part by consistent attention to fitness.

Efficiency and resistance to fatigue are both increased, and in an emergency such as a forced landing in the sea or at an isolated place, the chances of survival are much greater in those who possess energy reserves upon which they can call. Physical training may be dull and uninspiring if not properly conducted, and it is not easy to persuade members of aircrew to take part in it, but if its value is logically explained to them and the physical training which they are called upon to do is conducted in an interesting and entertaining way, they respond as sensible men do on seeing a probable advantage to themselves. The attitude that physical training bears no relationship to flying should be discouraged by showing how physical training builds up the general health and how in particular respects it helps to solve the unique problems associated with flying. It has been observed that a keen instructor, possessed of a sound knowledge and ingenuity in choosing the right type of exercise, can successfully persuade members of aircrew of the value of physical training and dissociate it in their minds from the activities of the parade ground. Short games, for example, volley ball, are of great value in developing quick eye movements and neuro-muscular reactions and in stimulating a competitive spirit, but whatever is done the instructor must take a personal interest in every member of his class and learn their individual needs and characteristics.

Constipation

Irregularities of the bowels, of which the commonest symptom is constipation, may be overcome to a greater or lesser extent by appropriate exercises. A strong abdominal wall not only prevents displacement of the stomach and intestines, but by its massaging effect also helps to maintain the tone of the involuntary muscle within their walls. Good habits are essential in promoting healthy functions of the bowels and they are most likely to be maintained by regular exercise.

Constipation is usually associated with the formation of gases within the bowel: at high altitudes these gases expand and may give rise to discomfort and pain. The gas is formed from the contents of the stomach and the small and large intestines, and although much can be done to prevent excessive formation of gas by avoiding unsuitable meals, a regular and thorough evacuation of the bowels every day is the best safeguard.

Cramp

Muscular cramp is probably caused by a local increase of lactic acid produced by muscle activity; it is more likely to occur when the limbs are cold and the vessels constricted, because then an adequate supply of oxygenated blood cannot reach the muscles. As already mentioned, the presence of oxygen is necessary for the removal of lactic acid. Cramp occurs in flying personnel when the circulation has been slowed down as a result of cold and inability to move the limbs. There are certainly other factors in the production of cramp, but cold and immobility are the most important.

The obvious means, therefore, of preventing cramp are the wearing of warm, loose clothing and exercise of the muscles. Stretching of the muscles is the best movement; exercise and comparatively simple movements can successfully mobilise the muscle fibres. For example, cramp in the small muscles under the foot or in the calf of the leg can usually be overcome by strong dorsiflexion of the foot in spite of the pain which this may cause. Cramp in the quadriceps or adductors may be overcome by flexing or abducting the leg. Cramp is less common in the upper limbs because their movements are less restricted.

The problem of cramp is closely associated with the need for muscular relaxation; tense, contracting muscles tire readily and it is important that no muscle during flight should be called upon to do more than its necessary portion of work. The problem is more psychological than physical; a tense, emotional state produces tense muscles, but much can be done by deliberate relaxing of the muscles and movement of their antagonists. After long operational trips airmen may suffer from nervous and muscular tension to such an extent that they find difficulty in sleeping. Despite fatigue the mind remains active, recapitulating the events of the day, and the muscles are kept in a state of tension instead of relaxing. Some benefit can be obtained by focusing the attention upon proper relaxation of the muscles. They are best relaxed by slow contractions of all the large muscle groups several times with attention to the antagonists, after which the limbs may be placed in the most comfortable position, usually the semiflexed position. A new attempt may then be made to go to sleep.

Skilfully performed, massage has a most soothing and beneficial effect, both physically and psychologically, upon the fatigued person and helps him to relax his muscles; it also helps to restore the circulation and dispel waste products from the tissues. Radiant heat is also of value as it produces dilation of the blood vessels in the affected part and increases the blood supply.

Lack of these facilities need be no deterrent; considerable relief can be obtained from unskilled massage provided it is applied steadily and rhythmically to the muscles only, with live oil or talcum powder as a lubricant. An electric stove may be used as a good substitute for a radiant heat lamp.

CHAPTER VI
GENERAL FITNESS

THE health of a individual depends to a large extent upon his personal habits, Good habits in relation to health should be acquired at an early age, so that they are practised automatically as age increases. Sound health is one of man's most valuable assets; the rules to preserve it are comparatively simple yet few people devote as much time and money to it as they spend on keeping their cars in good working order. A healthy body can only be acquired by a long term policy. The expectation of a rapid return for the expenditure of money or time leads to disappointment as far as the body is concerned. Physiological factors make constant attention necessary and unfortunately there are always difficulties such as lack of facilities for exercise in the fresh air, long working hours, and the many counter-attractions of life in a town.

The instructor, for his part, must pay special attention to his personal fitness. Instruction in physical training is work which requires considerable mental concentration as well as physical effort. The instructor must show a genuine keenness and enjoyment in his work thereby giving a lead to his class; this is only possible if he himself is feeling fit. To make a pretence of fitness is useless and is not likely to be convincing to the members of a class.

Some of the more important principles of general health which are applicable to physical training are described below.

Regularity of Habits

The body is a living mechanism which acts most efficiently when all its functions are performed regularly without strain. The first and most important rule of health is to be regular about times of eating, emptying the bowels, working and sleeping.

Irregularity in emptying the bowels is a very common fault, and is often the cause of constipation and digestive troubles; if the desire to defaecate is neglected, the walls of the rectum relax and the sensation disappears. Continuation of these bad habits causes distension of the rectal walls which lose their tone, and though a small amount of faeces may be passed each day, much remains in the rectum. A good all round diet with plenty of fruit and vegetables a glass of water in the early morning, and exercise, help to correct constipation; but it is most important that a regular time preferably after breakfast, should be allotted for defaecation, and that the habit of emptying the bowels at this time should be established.

The Value of Sunlight

The play of air and sunlight upon the bare skin is invigorating and produces a tonic effect upon the whole body. The action of air currents improves the skin circulation and is just as beneficial as sunlight. Certain rays emitted from the sun, called ultra-violet* rays, provide most of the health-giving properties of sunlight.

The practice of sunbathing is only beneficial if the time of exposure and the area of skin exposed is increased gradually over a period of ten days or more. People who bask in a sunny corner can tolerate less than those who are engaged in some form of manual work or exercise.

Ventilation

In a crowded room the air is continually being deprived of its oxygen, while carbon dioxide is being added to it. Nevertheless, even in an ill-ventilated room, sufficient oxygen is always present to supply the needs of the persons within it. It is the change in physical rather than chemical properties of air which is responsible for the feeling of discomfort in an ill-ventilated room. The air is overheated, moist and stagnant. In such an atmosphere the body cannot give out its heat in the normal way; but if there is a moving current of relatively cool air, even though it may not be fresh air, body heat can be given out and no feeling of discomfort is produced.**

The problems of ventilation become of greatest importance during the winter when weather conditions make it necessary for work to be carried on indoors. Unfortunately ventilation is not a subject to which architects have paid enough attention until recent years and there are consequently still many buildings in which it is inefficient or non-existent. The realization that poor ventilation leads to mental and physical inefficiency and therefore to financial loss by reduction in working hours, has recently stimulated interest in this important subject.

The object of ventilation is to make rooms or buildings comfortable and healthy to work in by maintaining a good circulation and exchange of air within them and by keeping the air at an even and suitable temperature. Cold air coming in through the window, being heavier than the warm air inside,

* They are called ultra-violet because their position in the spectrum is beyond that of the violet rays.

** The pressure of the oxygen in the atmosphere of the most crowded room is greater than that exerted by the oxygen in the atmosphere at 5,000 ft. above sea level, a level at which many health resorts are situated.

The 146 persons imprisoned in the Black Hole of Calcutta did not die from lack of oxygen but from the effects of overheating.

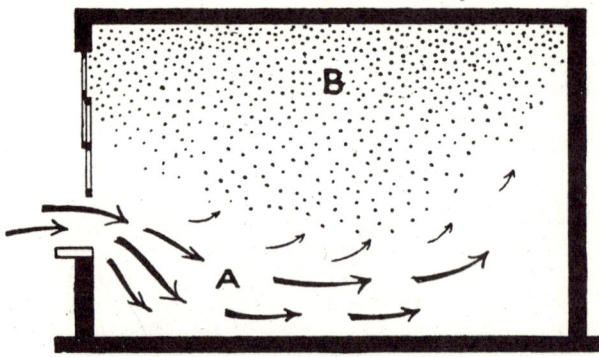

FIGURE 145—Diagram showing currents of cold air entering through sash window opened at the bottom only
A—Cold currents of air
B—Warmer air not being circulated

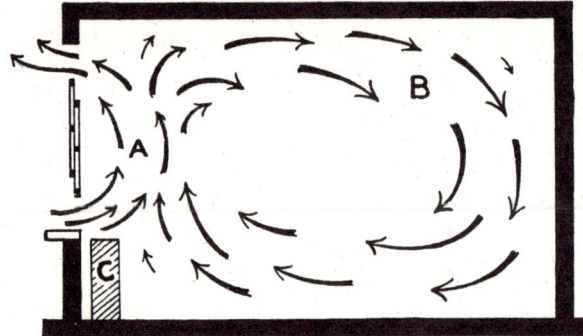

FIGURE 146—Diagram showing the effect of a radiator and the opening of the upper part of the window
A—Currents of air warmed by radiator
B—Warm air circulating more freely
C—Radiator

immediately flows along the floor displacing the warmer air upwards (Figure 145); but if there is a radiator in front of the window, the air entering from outside is suitably warmed, whereupon it rises and then descends near the centre of the room when it cools (Figure 146).

Cold downward draughts near the window cannot be prevented in a room in which there are no radiators or other form of heating near the window.

It is important to remember that sash windows should always be opened at the top, for this makes possible the escape of the warmer and vitiated air which collects in the upper part of the room. If windows are opened both at the top and the bottom, so much the better, if it is not too cold, because this facilitates a good circulation of air.

The Effects of Alcohol

The effects of alcohol upon the body are summarized in the Report of the Royal Commission on Licensing 1931.

(1) Alcohol is primarily a drug acting directly on the nerve centres.

(2) The action of alcohol is essentially narcotic* and not stimulant.

(3) Alcohol taken in excess may exert, like any other drug, a poison action; and if taken habitually in excess may cause or contribute to a variety of diseases.

(4) The drug or poison action of alcohol is substantially restricted when alcohol is taken in dilute solution or with food.

(5) Alcohol has certain food, or fuel, value, the scope of which, however, is strictly circumscribed by the disadvantages of its drug action.

* Narcotic means 'inducing drowsiness or insensibility.'

(6) The use of alcohol as an aid to work whether physical or mental, is physiologically unsound.

(7) Alcohol has no curative or prophylactic* properties, although within a strictly limited range of conditions, it has a certain therapeutic value.

Smoking

There is now evidence that cigarette smoking, even in moderation, is deleterious to the health. The smoking of over twenty cigarettes a day is very likely to interfere with the normal working of the digestive and respiratory passages. Nicotine, among other physiological effects, has a depressant action on the appetite and the smoke irritates the membrane lining the respiratory passages, giving rise to chronic bronchitis and to a greater liability to cancer of the lung in later life.

There is undoubtedly a large psychological factor which makes smoking such a popular habit and excessive smoking is often associated with other undesirable habits such as the failure to take regular or adequate meals and to get sufficient sleep. The use of tobacco is commonly supposed to be a cure for 'nervousness' but, so far from being a nerve sedative, excessive smoking may actually promote nervous signs and symptoms.

The Spread of Infection

Infectious diseases are spread from one person to another by germs which are living micro-organisms so small that some cannot be seen even with a high-powered microscope. Not all germs are harmful; some perform a most important function in agriculture and industry. The large intestine always contains billions of germs which have no deleterious effect upon the body, and some have a beneficial effect.

Germs gain access to the body by inhalation, through the various orifices of the body or through a break in the skin. When infectious diseases are spread by inhalation, the germs of an infected person are conveyed in small droplets of moisture expired in the breath; thus when a person coughs or sneezes, the droplets and the germs contained in them are projected a distance of five or six feet into the air. In a crowded room where the air is quite motionless, the droplets may be inhaled by a person in such concentrations that he becomes infected. The liability to infection is increased in damp weather because the droplets remain suspended in the air longer before they ultimately fall to the ground. Diphtheria, scarlet fever, measles and tuberculosis can be spread by droplet infection.

A curious bacteriological fact is the ability of some persons to carry virulent germs about in their nose or throat apparently without suffering any ill effects; these people are called *carriers* and have developed their own immunity, but if the germs are transferred to another person, the disease which the particular germ causes, may develop in a severe form; examples are tonsillitis, scarlet fever and diphtheria.

Tonsillitis, scarlet fever and diphtheria may also be spread by drinking infected milk, if the milk is consumed without boiling or pasteurization; tuberculosis and undulant fever may be transmitted in the same way. Typhoid, which is a disease mainly affecting the intestines, is contracted by drinking milk or water which has been contaminated by typhoid germs. The dairy man who has a mild form of typhoid, without any obvious symptoms, may contaminate the milk supply to a whole town by lack of cleanliness in his personal habits.

The body has a certain amount of resistance to all types of germs. The germs which cause pneumonia can often be found in the throat but unless the person becomes run down or is exposed to a severe chill, they seldom cause disease. The body can cope with a certain number of germs but if the concentration is too great, infection eatablished itself.

* Prophylactic means 'having a preventive action.'

The knowledge of how disease is spread ought to enable us to avoid it to a large extent, by taking the necessary precautions. Unfortunately people have a habit of treating the common cold and the milder forms of infectious disease, such as influenza, in a lighthearted way and of carrying on with the day's work even with a slight fever. The individuals who decided to carry on when they know that they are not fit to do so, are acting selfishly, not only by prolonging their own infection but by spreading their germs to others who may be much more susceptible than themselves.

Prevention of Infection

The onus of preventing the spread of infection naturally rests on the infected individual at first; if he delays seeing a medical officer and continues at his work, he is likely to infect others. If he must cough or sneeze in public places, he should do so into a handkerchief, 'Coughs and sneezes spread diseases' is true and good propaganda.

A person who leads a healthy life with as much fresh air, sunshine and exercise as possible, with sufficient sleep and a reasonable diet, has a greater resistance to disease than one who does not. Fresh air is beneficial in that it is comparatively pure compared with the atmosphere of a stuffy room which contains many millions of germs and dust particles which, when inhaled, have to be dealt with by the various germ-resisting mechanisms of the body; if this mechanism is overworked, infection is more likely to gain a footing.

Acclimatization of the Body to Exposure

Warfare requires fitness from those actively engaged in fighting, of a type which not only enables them to withstand physical fatigue but also exposure to extreme climatic conditions. Airborne troops particularly are likely to be exposed to such conditions and they must therefore be trained to fend for themselves in all circumstances.

The process of increasing the body's resistance to exposure is a physiological one; it can only take place gradually. To acquire ordinary physical fitness by means of athletic training is an easier and a shorter process.

Cold and wet weather are the chief enemies of troops who are compelled to bivouac in open, unprotected ground. The cold is intensified by damp clothing, because the clothes lose their normal insulating action and the heat is more rapidly conducted away from the body by their moisture. It is the aim in training airborne troops, to harden them so that they can sleep under such circumstances. Sleep is essential and without it physically fatigued troops become completely exhausted within 48 hours.

The average person who leads a comparatively sheltered life can maintain a normal body temperature only within narrow limits, because the centre in the brain which regulates temperature has never been called upon to make adjustments to meet extremes of heat and cold. The capacity to increase resistance to extreme temperatures is nevertheless present and if it is developed at an early age, the body can become extraordinarily hardened to exposure.

The body derives its heat from the muscles and the digestive organs; during activity the muscles are by far the larger source of heat, by reason of their conversion of chemical substances into energy. When the body is at rest the muscles are in a state of reduced tone and are therefore producing only a small amount of heat.

The amount of heat provided by the digestive organs also fluctuates and is greatest during active digestion. The appetite is increased during cold weather to provide heat both during digestion and muscular activity. A meal at night before sleep can prevent chill by providing heat from the digestive processes at a time when the activity of the muscles is at its lowest. For this reason airborne troops are instructed to try to have a meal at the end of the day.

In cold weather the heat regulating centre in the brain helps to keep up the body tempertaure by reducing the amount of heat lost from the skin; this is effected by the contraction of the superficial blood vessels so that only the minimum requirements of blood reach the skin. On a cold day the hands are sometimes red and cold, or even blue, because complete contraction of the small arteries and an incomplete contraction of the venous ends of the capillaries has occurred. The result is a stagnation of blood in the capillaries, the blueness being due to the de-oxygenation of the blood.

If the body temperature reaches a subnormal level, we increase the output of heat from muscular work by shivering.

Most civilized races wear more clothing than is necessary to maintain normal body temperatures. Overclothing reduces resistance to exposure and is unhealthy because it does not allow fresh air to come into contact with the skin. Airborne troops are conditioned by gradually discarding clothing until they are accustomed to wearing only the minimum necessary to prevent the body from being uncomfortably cold.

There is no doubt at all as to the effectiveness of this hardening process, but it must be carried out gradually. A long distance swimmer does not suffer from fatigue so much as from cold, and it is only by training his heat regulating mechanism as well as his muscular system that he can successfully withstand the effects of cold. Negro races can withstand the tropical sun and the cold tropical night equally well, not because they have a special inherited resistance but because their bodies have become accustomed to wide variations in temperature since childhood. The white races have a similar latent capacity for acquiring immunity to exposure, but under civilized conditions it is never developed to any extent except in special circumstances.

The success of the hardening process carried out on a grand scale during the recent war is a good illustration of the great powers od adaptation possessed by the body.

CHAPTER VII
MEDICAL REHABILITATION

MEDICAL rehabilitation is the process whereby an individual who has suffered disablement from any cause, is restored to a state in which he is able to function again as an active member of the community. This, in the Service, fits him for the full or limited duties of his branch and in civil life enables him to earn his living without dependence upon charitable organizations or compensation payments. It is a process of mental and physical reconditioning which begins when the patient is admitted to hospital and finishes when he is back at suitable work.

In the Royal Air Force the treatment of the disabled patient can be divided into three stages, the first spent in hospital, the second at a rehabilitation unit, and the third in finding proper employment. Not every patient who is admitted to a hospital goes through all three stages; some are discharged to their unit straight from hospital and a high percentage at rehabilitation units never present any problem of disposal as they are made fit to return to full duties.

The Rehabilitation Unit

A rehabilitation unit provides the necessary extra treatment required after discharge from hospital for those cases still unfit to return to their former work, the interval between the discharge from hospital and the return to work thus being bridged. There is no interruption in treatment and it is carried on from the same stage which had been reached in hospital and is continued until maximum function is regained. When a patient recovers sufficient function to perform his previous work, he is discharged to his unit either with or without limitations, but if, after a fair trial at a rehabilitation unit, it is evident that a patient is not going to make a sufficiently good recovery to enable him to perform his previous work, he is either discharged to take up a new form of employment or is sent to another type of rehabilitation unit where he can learn a trade of his own choice, suited to his particular disability.

The aim of a rehabilitation unit is to restore the patient to his maximum capacity for work in the shortest possible time. The longer a patient is under treatment, the more time he has to worry about his disability and his prospects of recovery.

The successful achievement of this aim depends largely on team work, the team consisting of the medical officer as head of the team, the physical fitness officer, the occupational therapist, the physiotherapist, the physical training instructor (or remedial gymnast), the technical training instructor, the welfare officer, and the patient. The team provides the guidance and supervision during treatment, while the patient must co-operate to the best of his ability, remembering always that the recovery of good function finally depends upon his own personal efforts.

The amount of accommodation and remedial apparatus varies considerably in different units. It is, of course, advantageous to have plenty of gymnasium space and large playing fields but they are not essential; much can be done by improvization.

A cheerful atmosphere is a necessary part of treatment. A patient who has spent three or four months in bed or in a plaster is apt to be depressed by the monotony of his existence and a little apprehensive about his ultimate recovery. It is the duty of the staff to prevent such an outlook by creating an optimistic spirit and a desire to get well among all patients. Once a good atmosphere is established, the instructor's work becomes much easier, for the patient does not need to be coaxed in his exercises; instead he enjoys performing them and his enjoyment increases the benefit derived from them. Furthermore, new patients arriving from hospital, who see their fellow patients' enthusiasm and confidence, are readily stimulated to make new and greater efforts to speed their own recovery.

Organization

The organization of rehabilitation units in the Royal Air Force is generally similar though it varies in detail. Each unit is divided for the purpose of remedial activities into several main divisions according to disability. For example, one division may consist of lower limb injuries and another of purely medical cases, such as patients recovering from pneumonia or general debility. Each main division is subdivided into classes, the activities of which are suitably graded for the particular disability. Thus it may be seen that the patient will progress from an early class with a reduced amount of mobility to later classes with more mobility, all the time being encouraged by progression through the classes and competition between members in the class.

On arrival, and once a week thereafter, each patient is interviewed by the medical officer who makes a note of the clinical condition and decides upon the programme of treatment. The P.T. instructor is always present at the weekly clinics to discuss the progress of the patient and to arrange any changes of treatment. The programme for each patient is individually prepared by the medical officer at the first interview and this may involve any of the members of the rehabilitation team. The daily programme is divided into half-hourly treatment periods and these are arranged according to a set pattern for each class to allow sufficient periods for relaxation, and variety in exercises and remedial games.

Specimen Programme for Early Stages

0830—0845	Suitable warming-up exercises, breathing exercises, short walk.
0845—0915	Remedial exercises.
0915—0945	Break
1015—1045	Remedial exercises.
1045—1115	Remedial games.
1115—1200	Swim; minor games such as quoits or badminton.
1200—1400	Lunch.
1400—1430	Remedial exercises.
1430—1500	Remedial games.
1500—1530	Break.
1530—1630	Walk, swim, cycle ride, etc.

All the remedial exercises should, in the early stages, be conducted individually rather than in a class.

Each patient is allotted to a basic class and the daily routine altered according to the needs of the individual patient, some treatment periods being used by other members of the rehabilitation team. In this way a varied programme may be arranged to suit every disability and patient.

In addition to the above, lectures of general interest and trips to the theatre, cinema, local beauty spots, etc., are included to prevent monotony, maintain morale, and encourage the wish for recovery.

ROLES OF THE REHABILITATION TEAM

Medical Officer

The medical officer initiates all treatment for patients and guides their progress through the classes. He co-ordinates and varies the daily programme of the patient according to his progress and he finally decides fitness for duty or civil employment.

Physical Fitness Officer

This officer supervises the activities of the P.T. instructors in their classes and ensures that the correct class routines are adhered to and that the exercises are given in accordance with the medical officer's requirements.

Occupational Therapist

This member of the team has three main tasks:—
  (i) The use of various crafts to produce specific muscle movements with a view to increasing their co-ordination, power and efficiency. Repetitive exercises may be given without fear of boredom because the patient produces an article of use as the result of his labours, *e.g.* carpentry, weaving, basket work.
  (ii) The supervision of the methods by which the normal functions of daily living may be acquired in disabled patients. For instance, the use of springs to allow a patient to eat who has weak shoulder or elbow muscles.
  (iii) The design and production of splints and gadgets to assist in (ii) above.

Physiotherapist

In the physiothrapy department patients receive individual attention to replace class work wholly or in part where groups class work may not or cannot be effective. The physiotherapist makes use of heat, light and electrical means to assist in individual treatments. In this department individual muscle build-up and passive movements may also be used. This is the only department in which passive treatments may be given to a patient; in all other departments the treatment is one of activity on the part of the patient.

Physical Training Instructor (or Remedial Gymnast)

The physical training instructor at a rehabilitation unit has received a basic training in anatomy, physiology and pathology before he is qualified to take part as a member of the rehabilitation team. Each instructor may have a class of 15 to 30 patients and each patient must be regarded by him as an individual problem.

It has been seen how the instructor is responsible for a particular class throughout the day in its routine treatment. He must supervise the exercises and give individual instruction where necessary. He must know the diagnosis and the more important features of the history and treatment of each patient in his group. He should know the patients personally and make them realize that he is interested in their recovery. It is essential to gain their confidence to make the remedial exercises of real value. In this way the instructor maintains continuous supervision over the activities of his patients and is able to supply valuable information to the medical officer about a patient's psychological background from sustained personal observation.

It can be seen from the above that the physical training instructor is a most valuable member of the team.

Technical Training Instructors

Where technical tradesmen are being rehabilitated not only must the physical treatment of the patient be considered but also the ability to perform the duties of his trade. If treatment is prolonged, skills may be lost and theory clouded. By making technical training instructors and equipment available, skills may be recovered and work ability tested to ensure fitness to return to the original job prior to discharge. Where disability makes this impossible, advice may be given about skills which may be developed in an allied trade or about ability to perform a civilian trade.

Welfare Officer

No patient can be completely co-operative when worried, for example about family affairs or his future. The welfare officer is an essential confidante who can often make the path of rehabilitation smoother by suitable action. He is responsible for maintaining contacts with civilian bodies for the resettlement of disabled people and also for the organization of the trips and outings so necessary for those who may be having prolonged treatment.

PSYCHOLOGICAL FACTOR IN REHABILITATION

Medical rehabilitation involves the study of the whole man. Patients who have been under treatment for a long time require mental as well as physical reconditioning. The most expert treatment is much discounted whilst the patient is not mentally co-operative or has no will to recover. The will-power of the individual exerts a powerful effect upon his ultimate recovery.

The psychological reaction to physical disability varies considerably with the personality of the patient. Such reactions may, for convenience of description, be divided into three main categories.

First there are those people who are determined to make the best of the difficulties whatever they are; such individuals present no problem in treatment. Their presence at rehabilitaion units is of great assistance to both staff and patients, for by their keenness and example they give a lead to their fellow patients.

Secondly, there are those who react less favourably to disability and show less initiative in carrying out their activities than those in the first category.

This is largely due to a lack of self-confidence. Such persons are keen enough to overcome their disability but they require encouragement and supervision before they can be persuaded to make that extra physical and mental effort which is necessary. As soon as they have gained confidence in themselves, they make a good recovery or as good a recovery as their disability allows.

Thirdly, there are those, fortunately few in number, who present a combined psychological and physical problem. Such persons are emotionally unstable under normal conditions and often unduly anxious about their health, but when a physical disability is added their anxieties are increased to such an extent and their fear of permanent disability so exaggerated that a normal recovery of function is difficult without psychological help.

A patient who is not progressing as rapidly as his physical condition appears to warrant is probably kept back by psychological factors. He may feel uncertain of himself and his capacity to earn a living under competitive conditions, and be unable to face realities. As long as this uncertainty is present in his mind, he escapes the difficulties ahead by unconsciously prolonging and exaggerating his disability. The patient genuinely believes that there is something abnormal about his particular disability and becomes quite indignant if it is suggested that he is imagining his symptoms; this is a form of mental illness called a *neurosis*. It is quite different from malingering which is a conscious simulation of disease; and is rarely seen.

These patients require sympathetic but firm handling; they are always a problem to both instructor and medical officer; they are unhappy individuals not mixing very much with other patients. They have a grievance and until that grievance is removed by providing them with a real incentive to get well, a good functional recovery is not likely to take place.

INDEX

	Page No.
ACCLIMATIZATION	148
Acetabulum	12
Achilles tendon	78
Acromion	9
Acromio-clavicular joint	21
Adam's apple	96
Adductor longus, magnus, and brevis	75
Afferent nerves	110
Agonists	113
Air passages	96
Alcohol, effects of	146
Anaemia	91
Anal canal	106
Antagonists	113
Anterior horn cells	115
Anterior tibial muscle	77
Aorta	94
Aponeurosis	41
Arches of the foot	15
Arteries	92
Astragalus (see Talus)	
Atlas	7
Auricles of the heart	94
Axis	7
Axons	108
BICEPS brachialis	60
Biceps femoris	75
Bicuspid valve	93
Bile duct	102
Blacking out	141
Blood, circulation of the	92
composition of	91
corpuscles	91
pressure	94
Body types	120
Bolus	104
Bone, structure of	1
types of	2
Brachialis	60
Brain	107
Breathing, varieties of	137
Bronchial tubes	96
CALCANEUS or heel bone	14
articulation of	14
Calf muscles	78
Calories	105
Cancellous bone	1
Capillaries	92
Carbohydrates	103
Carbon dioxide percentage in normal air	99

	Page No.
Carpus	11
Cartilage	1
Central nervous system	107
Cerebellum	112
Cerebrum	111
Cervical curve	4
Cervical vertebrae	4
Circulatory changes during exercise	95
Circumduction	22
Clavicle	9
Claw hand	67
Clothing	148
Coccyx	7
Colles fracture	25
Compact bone	1
Comparison of function in upper and lower limbs	27
Complemental air	99
Condyles	14
Condyloid joint	19
Constipation	143
Co-ordination of muscle action	113
Coracoid process	9
Coracobrachialis	61
Costal cartilage	8
Cramp	143
Cranial nerves	114
Cruciate ligaments	24
Cuboid bone	14
Cuneiform bones	14
DEAD space air	99
Defaecation	110
Deltoid	57
Dendrites	108
Diaphragm	39
Diet	102
Digestion	104
Dorsiflexion at ankle joint	26
at wrist joint	25
EFFECTS of 'g'	142
Efferent nerves	110
Energy requirements	105
Epiglottis	100
Eversion of foot	26
Exposure	148
External oblique muscle of abdomen	40
Extensors of the fingers and thumb	63
toes, long	77
wrist	64

	Page No.
FASCIA	73
Fatigue	140
Fats	103
Feet, defects of	133
Femur	14
Fibula	14
Fitness, factors influencing	144
Flexors of the fingers and thumb	62
toes, long	77
wrist	63
GASTROCNEMIUS	78
Glenoid fossa	9
Gluteus maximus	70
medius	71
minimus	71
Glycogen	116
Grey matter	108
Gullet	100
HAEMOGLOBIN	91
Hamstring muscles	75
Health, general	143
Heart, structure of	92
rate and output of	96
Housemaid's knee	165
Humerus	11
ILIACUS	69
Ilium	12
Infection	147
Infraspinatus	59
Inguinal ligament	41
Innominate bone	12
Insertion of muscle	29
Intercostal muscles	39
Internal oblique muscle of abdomen	42
Interossei	66
Intervertebral disc	4
Intestine	102
Inversion of the foot	26
Involuntary muscle	28
Involuntary nervous system	110
Ischium	12
JOINT, acromioclavicular	21
ankle	26
elbow	22
hip	25
knee	25
rib	21
sacro-iliac	12
shoulder	21
wrist	25

	Page No.
Joints, radius and ulna, between	22
types of	17
ball and socket	19
condyloid	19
gliding	19
freely movable	19
hinge	19
immovable	19
pivot	19
saddle	19
of the vertebral colum	19
KIDNEYS	106
Knee cap	12
Knee jerk	111
Kyphosis	121
LACTIC acid	116
Larynx	96
Lateral curvature of the spine	131
Latissimus dorsi	50
Levator ani	47
Levator scapulae	52
Lever action of muscles	29
Ligament	2
Liver	101
Longitudinal arch of foot	15
Longus colli	33
Lordosis	127
Lumbar curve	4
Lumbricals	66
Lungs	96
Lymphatic glands	92
MALLEOLUS	14
Marrow, bone	1
Massage	144
Mesentery	100
Metacarpals	11
Metatarsals	14
Micturition	111
Minerals, in diet	104
Motor nerve	110
Movements at the ankle joint	27
elbow joint	22
hip joint	25
knee joint	25
shoulder joint	21
wrist joint	25
between radius and ulna	22
Movements of the ribs	21
shoulder girdle	21
tarsus	26
thorax	21

	Page No.
Movements of the thumb	66
vertebral column	19
Muscle, actions, summary of	81
contraction	116
co-ordination	113
properties of	114
structure of	28
tendon	28
types of, involuntary	28
striped	28
unstriped	28
voluntary	28
Muscles, of posture	118
of the abdomen	40
foot	80
forearm	62
hand	66
lower limb	68
pelvis	47, 68
posterior abdominal wall	46
shoulder	57
shoulder girdle	49
spine	37
thorax	39
upper arm	60
upper limb	49
Muscle tone	113
Muscular fatigue	140
Mucous membrane	96
Mucus	96
NASAL passages	96
Navicular bone	14
Nerve, afferent	110
efferent	110
motor	110
peripheral	110
sensory	110
structure	108
Neurone	108
Neurosis	153
Nitrogen percentage in normal air	99
Nucleus of a cell	91
OCCUPATIONAL therapy	151
Olecranon	11
Origin of muscle	29
Os calcis (see calcaneus)	
Oxgen percentage in normal air	99
lack	99
absorption by haemoglobin	91
debt	116

	Page No.
PALMAR flexion	25
Parasympathetic nervous system	110
Patella or knee cap	12, 14
Pectoralis major	53
minor	54
Pelvic diaphragm	47
Pelvic girdle	12
Periosteum	1
Peripheral nerve	107
Peripheral nervous system	107
Peroneus longus	78
brevis	78
Phalanges	11
Pharynx	96
Plantar flexion	26
Plasma	91
Pleura	98
Pleural cavity	99
Posterior tibial muscle	78
Posture, muscles of	118
Pronation	23
Pronator quadratus	65
teres	65
Protein	91, 103
Psoas, muscle	68
Pubis	12
Pulmonary artery	94
circulation	94
vein	94
Pulse	94
Pylorus	100
QUADRATUS lumborum	46
Quadriceps	73
RADIAL deviation	25
Radius	11
Rectum	102
Rectus abdominis	44
Reflex arc	12
Rehabilitation centre	149
Relaxation	144
Residual air	99
Respiration, chemistry of	99
mechanism of	135
Reverse action of muscle	29
Rhomboideus major	52
minor	52
Ribs	3
Rickets	103
Rigid spine	131
SACRO-ILIAC joints	12
Sacrospinalis	37
Sacrum	7
Salivary glands	100

	Page No.		Page No.
Sartorius	73	Tensor fasciae latae	73
Scalene muscles	34	Teres major	59
Scaphoid	3	minor	59
Scapula or shoulder blade	2, 9	Thoracic breathing	137
Scoliosis	131	Thorax	8
Scurvy	103	Tibia	12, 14
Semimembranosus	75	Tidal air	99
Semitendinosus	75	Tone, muscle	113
Sensory nerve	110	Transverse arches of foot	15
Septum of nose	96	Transverse muscle of the abdomen	42
Serratus anterior	56	Trapezius	50
Sesamoid bones	31	Triceps	61
Shin bone or tibia	14	Tricuspid valve	93
Shivering	114	Trochanter	14
Shoulder girdle	9, 49	Tuberosity, greater	59
Sinuses, nasal	96	Tubules of kidney	106
Skin	106		
Smoking	147		
Sodium chloride in diet	106	Ulna	11
in sweat	107	Ulnar deviation	25
in urine	106	Ultra violet rays	145
Soleus	78	Unstriped muscle	28
Spinal chord	108	Ureter	106
Spine of scapula	9	Urethra	47
Splenius capitis	35		
Splenius cervicis	35		
Sternomastoid	32	Valves in the heart	94
Sternum	8	veins	92
Stomach	100	Veins	92
Subscapularis	59	Ventilation	145
Summary of muscle actions	81	Ventricle	94
Sunlight	145	Vertebra, cervical	4
Superficial muscles, illustrations of	84–90	dorsal	7
Supination	23	lumbar	7
Supinator, long	65	typical	2, 5
short	65	Vertebral column	3
Supplemental air	95	Vital capacity	99
Supraspinatus	59	Vitamins	103
Sweat glands	106	Vocal chords	96
Sympathetic nervous system	110	Voluntary or striped muscle	28
Synergists	113		
Synovial membrane	19	Water in the diet	103
Systemic circulation	92	Water on the knee	26
		White blood corpuscles	91
Talus	14	White matter of the nervous system	108
Tarsus	14	Windpipe	96
Tendon	28	Wrist drop	64